THE HOSPICE
VOLUNTEER HANDBOOK

THE HOSPICE VOLUNTEER HANDBOOK

VOLUME ONE -
THE FRIENDLY VISITOR

▲ ▲ ▲

Craig O. Lynch

ISBN # 1545215138
ISBN 13: 9781545215135

Library of Congress Catalog Number: 2017905552
CreateSpace Independent Publishing Platform
North Charleston, South Carolina

TABLE OF CONTENTS

From the Author ...

▲ ▲ ▲

"I HAVE WORKED AS A *Hospice Volunteer for over seven years with five dif-ferent Hospice Agencies in northern California. These have included Pathways Home Health and Hospice (South San Francisco), Gift of Love (Pacifica), Hospice of the Central Coast (Monterey), Vitas Healthcare and Hospice (Walnut Creek) and Hospice of the East Bay (Pleasant Hill). During this time, I had the profound privilege of spending time with well over 200 Individuals struggling with life-threatening disease. This also included interacting with many Family Members and close Loved Ones during this ordeal. I have also worked in the difficult and intense arena of Grief and Bereavement support for Survivors.*

"I also integrated these on-going activities with pursuing formal academic education concerning End-of-Life issues. I finally earned my Master's Degree from San Francisco State in 2012. My degree was granted in the Gerontology / Social Wok Department. My final Thesis was titled "Quality-of-Life Assessment of End-of-Life Care in American Healthcare Systems". During my extended time at SSF, I also did in-depth research in the areas of the Biology of Aging, Institutional Elder Care, Bio-Medical Ethics in Elder and End-of-Life Care, Public and Private Healthcare Systems, Public Healthcare Policy Development and Geriatric Nursing.

"Also during this time, I worked as a Social Services Specialist at three different Skilled Nursing Facilities (SNF). Each of these facilities housed up to 149 Residents, including those in permanent, custodial care, those

in temporary rehabilitation support as well as those in memory or dementia care. Within each of these challenging sectors, dealing with Patients facing a life shortening illness was always an on-going issue.

"This Handbook reflects and embodies the totality of these experiences."

FORWARD

▲ ▲ ▲

"I'M A HOSPICE VOLUNTEER...FACING THE PATIENT"...

"I'M HERE WITH YOU BECAUSE You are now facing the most chaotic and desperate Human challenge You will ever encounter. In all the myriad blinding courses of Human things, there is nothing so daunting as confronting one's own mortality. Even though You and I are different and unique People, as Humans we share a common bond, a common experience, a common history. We share common beginnings, process and destiny. I'm here because I feel terrible sympathy for my fellow Human Beings as they suffer. It is so very difficult to watch others endure disease, pain, incapacity, anguish, fear, confusion, injustice, uncertainty, loss of physical control, meaninglessness and an overwhelming sense of the inevitable loss of Self. So, I'm here to do the only possible thing I'm capable of doing. I pledge to bring my common Human self to be with You during your final journey. Together, we'll strive to maintain your inherent Dignity and Autonomy and Value as a Human Being so long as You live. I offer You my presence, my companionship, my time, my attention, my compassion and my heart. I have no ability to lead You on your journey, but I will try to remain at your side. I offer You one solemn promise. I will do my very best to insure that You will not perish from this world without another Human Heart beating at your side. I have no idea if this will somehow help You. But, I'm willing to try. For me, not trying is unthinkable. I tell You up front, that I have many stupid Human weaknesses and limitations. I do not possess the wisdom nor the power nor the virtue to alter the inevitable course of your debility and dying. I harbor no wise answers or comments or observations or insights for You. I cannot mend any broken relationships from Your past. I have no capacity to resolve your personal existential or private spiritual dilemmas. Any specific answers or resolutions You might discover during this tumultuous journey can only come from deep inside You. However, my being merely Human is hopefully what makes my presence here worthwhile. We can spend time together reminiscing, laughing, and crying. You can tell me about your youth, your family, school, work, interests, joys, successes, failures, regrets and the People who are most important to You. If You wish, You can explain to me your most profound valuations and ideals and assumptions about the life You are living. Or, we can spend time in complete silence. Together we'll try to spend this most precious time dwelling on whatever You find most significant. In retrospect, we might come to realize that every passing mundane moment in our routine lives has been far more profound and meaningful than we have ever dared to recognize. We might come to understand that every Human life consists of an endless series of miracles that we all too often overlook. I hope that in some meager way I ease your burden. You enrich my life more than I can possibly say. My greatest regret is that throughout all the countless stars and galaxies, You are utterly unique. When You finally vanish, there will never again be another You. And, when you are finally gone, I will once again shudder at what I fear is the terrible futility of my efforts to have somehow helped You during your most desperate days. Whether I actually helped or not, I will never be able to know for certain. And then, I will shed a tear in solitude and I will carry a new secret wound deep in the recesses of my silent and all too feeble Human heart. I am not sure how many more of these secret wounds I can endure. But I will often reflect back on the rare and rarified privilege You have given me, take a deep breath and then endeavor to carry on with the next Person...I'm a Hospice Volunteer"...

PROLOGUE

▲ ▲ ▲

"AFTER 7 YEARS AS A HOSPICE VOLUNTEER, I'VE LEARNED"...

* That our personal anguish, grief, confusion, anger or sense of injustice over watching the death of a cherished Loved One is ultimately the Human cost we pay for loving others; that in the myriad course of Human things, if we live long enough and love others deeply enough, we will inevitably suffer sorrow and grief.

* That in the depth of our grieving, we sometimes wonder if the price for loving others is simply too great of a personal Human cost; but, as time slowly passes, in the end we come to the rarified realization that we would not have it any other way; it is always and only the People in our lives that matter most.

* That once we take on the duties and activities of caring for Individuals struggling with a terminal disease, our personal lives will never be the same; that the long-term impact on us is both profound and permanent.

* That confronting Human mortality forces us to continually reexamine our deepest valuations and assumptions about our own Human lives and those we share our lives with; we tend to be driven towards a stark clarity about what matters most to us.

* That every single passing mundane moment in our Human lives is a gift that should be treasured; that our lives and the lives of those

around us are miraculous and exquisite, and yet at the same time, terribly fragile and tenuous.

- That we too often take these passing moments for granted; that our involvement in our daily lives is often lackadaisical and we are routinely obsessed with trivial or unimportant things.
- That our most precious and meaningful experiences are grounded in the People and relationships in our life; not in "things" such as money, houses, jewelry, fame, power or trophies; that when we or our Loved Ones are facing a life-threatening condition, our greatest sorrow centers around the terrible sense of loss of our closest Loved Ones and our relationships with them; that this is true whether our complex relationships are positive or negative.
- Ultimately, we realize that our sorrow and grief will fade, even though the desolate emptiness in our heart over losing a Loved One will never vanish.
- Yet, dying and death are an inherent part of the life cycle. This inevitability often causes Humans to ponder some of the most difficult and lofty questions ever conceived. This can include struggling with such issues as God, suffering, ignorance, justice, faith, eternity, transcendence, soul, destiny, and meaningfulness. Humans are compelled to reaffirm or reexamine their deepest assumptions about many of these specific subjects.
- How effectively Individuals manage this process has a profound impact on how they cope with the remainder of their lives and impending mortality.
- *People often ask me "WHY' I do such things. My reply is that is that if that seems to be a valid question to them – then there is no meaningful response for them.*
- *People also ask me "HOW" can I do such things. My answer is that if not me (and other Volunteers), then who will take on such challenges.*

I've also learned that the Learning never ends!

You as a Hospice Volunteer

▲ ▲ ▲

Basic Definitions

Hospice Care

HOSPICE CARE IS A COMPREHENSIVE approach of compassionate support for Individuals facing a life-threatening disease. As such, it is designed to encompass caring for the entire Human Person. This includes the physical, cognitive, emotional, social, spiritual and existential aspects of daily experiences. Each of these complex and varying dimensions are addressed by an "Interdisciplinary Team" or "Interdisciplinary Group" of professionals. An individualized Hospice "Plan of Care" is developed to provide on-going pain and symptom management or "comfort care" rather than specific treatments aimed at "curing" any underlying disease. Hospice does not seek to slow down nor hasten the natural dying process. Ideally, Patients are maintained within their primary "home setting" for as long as possible. Close Family Members and willing Loved Ones are trained by Hospice personnel to perform many aspects of routine daily care. Registered Nurses and Home Health Aides also provide regularly scheduled hands-on care and on-going assessment. Spiritual Counselors, Social Workers, Volunteers and various other specialized care providers are also available. Physician and nursing support is available 24/7 as needed. In order for an Individual to qualify for Medicare Hospice benefits, two Physicians must certify that the sick Patient is not expected to live longer than six months, assuming the primary disease runs its expected course. Following the death of the Patient, Hospice also then provides Grief and Bereavement Support to surviving Family Members and Loved Ones as needed. <u>The overall objectives in Hospice are designed to sustain or enhance the daily Quality-of-Life of the Patient, as well as surrounding Family and Loved Ones, over the course of the dying process.</u>

PALLIATIVE CARE

<u>Palliative Care is likewise a comprehensive approach of compassionate support for Individuals facing a life-threatening disease, as well as those suffering with severe chronic conditions.</u> The basic principle is that "comfort care" is the most effective strategy in coping with these challenging situations. It is generally a specialized form of care provided within a hospital setting and administered by hospital Staff. (Although there are some exceptions, the majority of Palliative Care programs in hospitals do not routinely use outside Volunteers.) It is likewise designed to provide the "best care possible" for the total Human Person. The on-sight Palliative Care Team endeavors to address the physical, cognitive, emotional, social, spiritual and existential aspects of daily experiences, as necessary. "Comfort care", including effective pain and symptom management are the central focus of daily efforts. Within a Palliative Care setting, further treatment protocols to effect potential "cures" of any serious diseases are not completely ruled out. The basic approach in Palliative support is comfort care on an on-going basis even while aggressive procedures designed to cure an underlying condition may still be considered. Patients being supported through Palliative Care do not need to "qualify" for medical benefits with a limited life expectancy of six months or less, as is required for Hospice benefits through Medicare or Medicaid. Financial support for most Palliative Care Patients within a hospital setting are usually provided through regular Medicare Part A, or through private insurance or resources. Again, similar to Hospice

care, <u>Palliative Care is ideally designed and administered to sustain the daily Quality-of-Life of both Patient and all surrounding concerned Loved Ones.</u>

▲ ▲ ▲

Like You, many Individuals in the United States may know something about Hospice Care. Unfortunately, for most this understanding is often limited and confusing. Many people have vague assumptions about Hospice being a "place" in a hospital or facility where terminally ill people go to die. Hospice is usually thought of as a form of medical or psychological support for Individuals when all hope for a "cure" has been exhausted. It is sometimes viewed as a consequence of "medical failure". The common presumption is that all that remains is a passive form of "comfort care", where nature is simply allowed to take its inevitable course. The dominant attitude with most People in the United States is that Hospice is a form of finally "giving up" or "quitting" in the face of an overwhelming and intractable disease. For many Individuals, these are compelling reasons to resist Hospice Care for themselves or a Loved One struggling with a serious illness.

Similar to many others, You may have become aware of Hospice support by being personally involved with the long-term illness and death of a Loved One or close Friend. Sadly, most Individuals are first exposed to the Hospice approach only when they are forced by personal circumstances to cope with a dying Loved One or Friend. You may well have witnessed Friends who have had to deal with their own Family or Loved Ones struggling with a terminal illness.

As an individual, your personal reasons to consider working in this intense arena are most likely as unique as You are. Everyone's history and experience and background are different. However, as with most forms of "volunteerism" in the society, the primary motivation cited by Individuals choosing to volunteer is an altruistic desire to "help others', to "give back to society" or to "contribute to noble or worthwhile causes or movements". Again, one of the most common reasons given by Hospice Volunteers for their involvement in the field is their personal experiences with a Hospice Agency while caring for a terminally ill Loved One. They witnessed first-hand the compassionate care and support and now seek to "help others" in a similar way.

In actuality, it does not matter what your personal motives are for becoming a Hospice Volunteer. Again, everyone is unique and everyone's reasons are valid. In the beginning, it does not matter what your personal beliefs or attitudes or expectations are concerning Hospice work. Your previous training and experiences are not terribly important. Your age and education are not critical factors. Like most people, You may well have endured struggles and disappointments and failures in your life. None of these issues will determine your effectiveness as a Hospice Volunteer.

It might be said that there are only three personal characteristics that are initially important for any Individual considering becoming a Hospice Volunteer. These include the following.

1. You must have a deeply caring and compassionate Human Heart with a genuine capacity for empathy and the sincere yearning to act on it. You generally feel that "true compassion demands action".
2. You must have both the desire and the courage to be willing to try to help a fellow Human Being struggling with a terminal illness. This will place You inevitably in close proximity to Human dying and death.
3. You must have an ability to be patient and reasonable with Yourself and to be motivated to continue to learn and grow and take on new challenges.

Beyond these three fundamental characteristics, the Volunteer Department of the National Hospice and Palliative Care organization (NHPCO) suggests a wider range of personal traits and experiences as being important for a Hospice Volunteer. These encompass the following factors.

- *Presence:* This is perhaps the most basic and yet meaningful form of Human caring for anyone with a terminal disease. It is simply the open willingness to offer full attention to such a fellow Human Being. This may be for several minutes or several hours. Such an encounter is especially powerful when verbal communication is no longer possible.
- *Ability to Listen Empathically:* This describes the uncommon ability to fully hear what another Person says without interruption, interpretation judgement or criticism. During the desperation and overwhelming circumstances of facing a terminal illness, most People long to be genuinely heard and understood.
- *Capacity for Calm and Comfort:* This entails the unique ability to remain serene and collected while engaged with another Person suffering a serious disease as well as surrounding Loved Ones.
- *Interpersonal Skills:* This encompasses the important talents, both natural and acquired, to interact with various types of Individuals in caring, meaningful and effective ways.
- *Caring and Compassionate:* This represents the essence of "why" Individuals choose to reach out to try to help another Human Being during times of great pain and sorrow. It is the inherent Human yearning to ease the suffering of others. This flows from an innate Human capacity to acknowledge and empathize with shared suffering and to respond to it.
- *Patience:* This encompasses the willingness to remain steadfast and dependable when working with Individuals struggling with their own debility and mortality.
- *Sensitivity:* This refers to the ability to be consciously mindful and respectful of another Person's stress and sorrow.
- *Courage:* This describes the basic emotional strength and willingness to deal with and persevere in the face of chaotic and difficult Human situations.
- *Personal Life Maturity and Life Experiences:* This encompasses the totality of a Person's growth and learning and acquired knowledge and understanding of the Human experience.

In practical fact, all but the very last component (*Personal Life Maturity and Life Experiences)* are abilities and skills that the Hospice Volunteer will gradually acquire over time by being involved with terminally ill Individuals and their Loved Ones.

▲ ▲ ▲

As a Hospice Volunteer, You will be engaged in an extraordinary and unique Human arena. You will be endeavoring to ease the burden of the most intense and desperate and profound Human experience there is. You will be cultivating the courage and patience to become a "companion along the way" to People in their journey towards imminent and inexorable mortality. Your compassionate "Co-Human presence" will be the most meaningful gift You can freely offer to a dying Person and to surrounding Loved Ones. You will be summoning the strength and self-discipline to be active in a field that most Individuals avoid even thinking about.   The emotional or existential benefits you might bring to Others can hardly be measured. To gently hold the hand of a dying Person may well be your greatest Human achievement. It may well transform You into the most important Human Being You will ever be.

At this point, You might well just be considering becoming a Hospice Volunteer. You may simply want to learn more about this challenging and rewarding field before You decide to become involved. Or, You may have already made the critical decision to engage in this work and are getting ready to take the initial training course offered by your Agency. You may have completed your training and are taking on your first assignments. Or, You may be a seasoned Volunteer with many profound and difficult assignments completed. No matter what stage You are at in this process, this book should be helpful to You for a variety of reasons.

How this Handbook is Organized

▲ ▲ ▲

This book is written specifically by a Hospice Volunteer for Hospice Volunteers. It is designed to help both new and experienced Volunteers. This "VOLUME I" Handbook focuses primarily on the "Friendly Visitor" roles and responsibilities within Hospice Care. It is the result of working for over seven years in this field, with five different Hospice Agencies. Most meaningful and profound is the fact that it is the reflection of sharing time with over 200 Patients coping with their own dying and death. It also encompasses the terrible and profound experiences endured by the Patients' surrounding Loved Ones.

Volunteers within this field will be asked to perform very specialized services. This Handbook is designed to guide and educate and assist Volunteers in these unique efforts. The Sections and Chapters in the book are organized to facilitate easy access to very specific subjects. This book does not need to be studied in any particular order. The theme of each Chapter can be chosen and reviewed by itself. So, e.g. if the aspiring or seasoned Volunteer has taken on a new Assignment to visit a Patient living permanently in a Skilled Nursing Facility or Nursing Home, Chapter Ten *"Patient Home Settings"* and Chapter Thirteen *"Volunteer Interaction with Patient and Family within various Home Settings"* should be informative and helpful. If as a Volunteer is asked to visit a Patient suffering with mild or severe cognitive decline, Chapter Sixteen *"Patients with Cognitive Deficits"* should prove extremely valuable. If a Volunteer goes on a first Respite Assignment, Chapter Fourteen *"Respite Visits"* can help.

The primary content of the Handbook is divided into six SECTIONS spanning nineteen Chapters.

SECTION I deals with a *"Hospice and Palliative Care Overview"*. These Chapters define the ideals and objectives of both Hospice and Palliative Care. They compare and contrast the two movements to each other. This includes their history, evolution, organization, regulatory control, personnel structure, delivery and payment systems, etc.

SECTION II encompasses *"Hospice and Palliative Care in American Society"*. These Chapters deal with the complex physical and psychological issues of Human aging over the Life Course and how they have changed dramatically over recent decades. Advancements in medicine and technology have completely altered the patterns of dying and death in modern American society. The Hospice and Palliative Care options within this context have gradually and yet begrudgingly emerged as an integral part of the overall healthcare arena.

SECTION III deals with *"Volunteer Preparation"*. *These Chapters* explain the various procedures and practical instructions Volunteers will be required to go through by the Agency before actually beginning work within the Hospice field. This includes Agency application, background check, TB test, etc. It also includes the basic Training required for Volunteer, such as the history and philosophy of Hospice, HIPAA requirements, Medicare, etc. It also details the process of exactly how Volunteers get started taking Assignments in the field.

SECTION IV describes *"Working with Patients – Loved Ones"*. The Chapters in this Section explore the many issues Hospice Volunteers may well deal with when interacting with Patients and Loved Ones during Assignments in the field. This includes descriptions of the Friendly Visitor's various roles, the types of encounters with Patients and Family, home settings and how they affect visitations, Respite and Vigil Assignments, cognitive issues and the behaviors and signs of approaching death. These issues can all be intense, chaotic, confusing and the more the Volunteer understands them, the more effective will be that Volunteer's interactions with Patient and Family Members.

SECTION V deals with *"Activities"*. These Chapters list specific practical suggestions about some of the Activities the Friendly Visitor might utilize when visiting a Patient. These include many types of Activities that range from very simple to very complex. A separate Chapter is devoted to the central activity of personal reminiscence. These guidelines are merely a set of possible suggestions the Volunteer can draw on as necessary.

SECTION VI surveys a list of *"Frequently Asked Questions"* concerning the Hospice Friendly Visitor Volunteer. This list focuses on practical, real-world issues that will certainly come up in the Volunteer's experience and growth.

Leading into each of the first five Sections are brief "Case Studies" which describe real-life Volunteer Assignments from the Author's own private files. The names and certain details have been altered to protect the full confidentiality of the Patients and Family Members involved. They were carefully chosen to illustrate a range of very typical visitation experiences.

▲ ▲ ▲

Author's Note: In writing this manuscript, I constantly tried to describe specific topics as clearly and concisely as possible. This was an on-going challenge, in that the Human issues and experiences explored in the book are immensely complex and varied among Individuals. However, for the sake of brevity and convention, I had to resort to certain terminology and generalized labels to cover subjects. I use the term *"Patient"* throughout the book to identify the "terminally ill Individual", the "dying Person", the "Person that is actively dying", the "Person certified as qualifying for Hospice Care" and even the "Hospice Person who died under Hospice Care". I do not like the term *"Patient"* as it seems to imply a cold, medicalized or clinical perspective toward the sick Person. This runs contrary to the Hospice and Palliative ideals of caring for the total Human Being, not simply addressing the disease. However, I chose to use the word *"Patient"* as the collective single term to identify the central Individual in End-of-Life Care rather than the multiple phrases listed above. I also used the terms *"Family"*, *"Family Members"*, *"Loved Ones"* and *"Close Friends"* throughout the book to describe a complex array of Individuals that may be associated with the Patient. Within a certain context, all of these terms or labels can be used to describe a single idea. Regardless of the exact connection these different individuals have with the Patient, in Hospice and Palliative Care, they can all be considered as having a significant Human relationship with the Patient. In other words, whomever the Patient regards as having an important and meaningful tie to the life of the Patient is ultimately regarded as *"Family"*. So, Family, Loved Ones and even Close Friends are within the critical social network of the Patient. Each Individual may play an integral part in the active care at the End-of-Life. Within the book, I also adopt the unconventional practice of "capitalizing" the "names" or "titles" of important Human Beings or subjects. This is simply an existential affirmation of my regard for the subjects and primary figures engaged in this most desperate and meaningful Human experience. As the Author I am solely responsible for any clumsy or inappropriate mistakes made in the manuscript.

COL

Hospice and Palliative Care Overview

▲ ▲ ▲

"You matter because you are you. You matter to the last moment of life, and we will do all we can not only to help you die peacefully, but also to live until you die."

Dame Cicely Saunders

"As a Hospice Volunteer, I've watched the subtle and ineffable mystery of being alive vanish from the eyes of a dying Human Being. How can there possibly be such wonder and beauty and complexity in one moment that somehow vanishes in the next. Perhaps I've stared into the abyss too many times."

COL

"...the approach and ideals of Hospice and Palliative Care have emerged as a hallmark of Human caring and dignity and reverence for the sanctity of Human Life during the most difficult of all Human experiences. No doubt, its powerful role as an integral part of a compassionate and effective healthcare system will only expand as time goes on."

COL

ALFRED

▲ ▲ ▲

I WAS ASKED BY THE Volunteer Coordinator at "Hospice of the East Bay" if I would be willing to take on a new assignment with a very challenging Patient. I was told that he was very strong willed and had actually "fired" a couple of previous Volunteers because he did not care for their company. I said I would give it my best shot.

Alfred was around 90 years old and lived in a private room in a very plush Assisted Living Facility in Pleasant Hill, California. He had several medical conditions that rendered him quite physically frail. He was a long-time diabetic, and had both respiratory and cardiovascular problems. However, he was very clear headed and active mentally. Over the course of our first several visits, he revealed an extraordinary life story and odyssey. Since I was always a history buff, I was fascinated with his narratives and was generally able to follow his storylines.

Alfred was born in Germany in the 1920s. He was a German Jew. As such, he experienced firsthand the plight of the Jewish community in Germany with the rise of the Nazi regime and vehement antisemitism. He spoke at length about being the object of ridicule and bigotry even as a young Jewish boy in a public school. He talked about how lonely and afraid he felt growing up in this environment. He had obviously carried the emotional impact of these early experiences throughout his entire life. He spoke dramatically about how "the Nazis killed his Mother" and he managed to escape with his Father and Brother to "Palestine" in the latter 1930s.

He finished growing into young adulthood while working in a small Jewish community located north of Tel Aviv. This is where he lived during the course of WW II. Although he did not go into a lot of detail, he said he was active with the revolt against the English and the conflicts with the Arab Palestinians during the 1948 Jewish revolution that led to the creation of the State of Israel.

He finally received the opportunity to immigrate to the United States and ended up in Wisconsin in the 1950s. He was taken in by a Jewish Cousin who had moved to the US several years earlier. There he got a great job "milking cows". He also met his future Wife who was coincidentally also a Jewish immigrant. Alfred then got the tremendous opportunity to continue his higher education. He actually went on to earn his PhD in Microbiology. He spent many years in research and then teaching in his chosen field. He eventually moved to Arizona and then finally to northern California where he retired. He and his Wife raised two sons. He also had several Grandchildren and a couple of Greatgrandchildren. His had led a remarkable life spanning a tumultuous history, living in several countries during extraordinary historical events and ended up with a prestigious career and extended family.

During most of our visits, he was intellectually animated and excited. In his room were many books about history, the state of Israel, WW II, Microbiology and other scientific subjects. He truly had a litany of stories to tell and relished in telling them. All I had to do was ask a specific question about a particular event or critical era and he was off and running. I always looked forward to our conversations.

However, there were several occasions during my visits when Alfred appeared to be very agitated or angry over what seemed to be recent or current circumstances. I tried to gently encourage him to tell me what was causing his distress. He alluded to specific issues with His two sons and how he felt he had been treated badly by them. It was very difficult for me to piece together what he was trying to say. His words and thoughts seemed to be somewhat disjointed and lacking focus.

On one such visit, I entered his room to discover one of his sons there. Alfred was acting very angry at him and complaining to him. I listened without saying anything and then afterwards spoke to his son outside the room for a few minutes. The son explained to me that Alfred was having more and more of these outbursts and that the family did not quite know what to do. They had been trying their very best to care for and support Alfred in recent years. Again, when I went back into the room and spoke with Alfred alone, he continued to express disapproval at his situation. I never did quite understand what he was so upset about when trying to explain it to me in private. Curiously enough, when I returned for subsequent weekly visits, Alfred was generally in good spirits, calm and not agitated and ready to discuss history, philosophy and science.

I visited Alfred over about eight weeks. Then, during my routine signing in at the lobby desk, I was told that Alfred had quite suddenly passed away the previous day. Even though he had been physically frail, it was somewhat of a surprise as he had been so active cognitively during recent visits. I still miss his lively spirit and extraordinary life stories.

CHAPTER 1

HOSPICE CARE

▲ ▲ ▲

WHEN YOU FIRST BEGIN WORKING as a Hospice Volunteer, the scope and objectives of Hospice Care within society may seem complex and even confusing. The Agency You start with will often seem to be very large with many different interacting departments. You will usually find yourself dealing with a variety of personnel with unique titles and responsibilities. Sometimes it is difficult to keep all these factors clear in your mind. Even after You complete the Agency Training Program, You may still have many questions. This Section is designed to expand your understanding of the basic principles and ideals of the Hospice approach to End-of-Life issues, so that You will be better equipped to understand your roles as a Volunteer.

In the United States, Hospice Care encompasses the following parameters.

* Hospice Care is a comprehensive approach of compassionate support for Individuals facing a life-threatening disease.
* The overall objective is to maintain or enhance the highest possible Quality-of-Life for the Patient during whatever time remains.
* Death is regarded as the natural conclusion to the overall Human Life Course. Hospice does not seek to disrupt the natural and inevitable process of dying. It does not endeavor to slow down nor hasten the End-of-Life.

- Hospice endeavors to address and care for the total Human Person, including medical, physical, emotional, social, spiritual and existential issues.
- The Agency will develop individualized strategy plans designed to provide on-going "comfort care", rather than treatment protocols aimed at "curing" any life-shortening or underlying disease.
- Pain management and symptom control are primary focuses within these care plans.
- A Hospice status generally requires two Physicians to agree that the Patient is not expected to live past six months, assuming the life-limiting disease runs its expected course.
- Hospice Care can be extended beyond the initial six months period with Physician recertification.
- A Patient can be removed from Hospice with an improved prognosis. Also, Patients are always afforded the autonomy of choosing to be removed from Hospice care if they so desire.
- Direct care and support are offered by an Interdisciplinary Team (IDT) or Interdisciplinary Group (IDG) of professionals, including Physicians, Case Managers, Nurses, Social Workers, Home Health Aides, Spiritual Councilors, and various Volunteers.
- Besides daily visits by Home Health Aids and routine visits by Nursing Staff and Volunteers, Physician and Nursing on-call support is offered 24 hours a day, 7 days a week by the Agency.
- Ideally, Hospice care is provided within the Patient's "home setting". This can include any Private Residence, Assisted Living Facility (ALF), Skilled Nursing Facility (SNF), Shelter or anywhere else. In severe cases, care can be extended into and integrated with Staff of a Sub-Acute Facility or an Acute Care Hospital.
- Ideally, within a private home setting, the daily hands-on "care unit" consists primarily of surrounding Family Members and Loved Ones. These "Informal Caregivers" are trained by the Agency Personnel to perform various daily tasks.

* Hospice services are generally fully paid for by Medicare, Medicaid (Medi-Cal in California) or private insurance. Hospice services are paid for by a specialized classification within Medicare Part A.
* Medicare stipulates 4 Levels of Hospice Care. These are "Routine Home Care", "Continuous Care", "General In-Patient Care" and "Respite/In-Patient Care". Each level encompasses different degrees of care and support and each is reimbursed at a different per-diem rate.
* Hospice agencies are required by Medicare, Medicaid and Medi-Cal to offer up to 12 months of Grief and Bereavement Support to surviving Family Members and Loved Ones, following the death of the Patient.
* Within a community, Hospice services are generally offered to anyone suffering a terminal disease. This includes Grief and Bereavement Support to anyone suffering the great personal loss of a Loved One. These services are offered regardless of an Individual's race, religion, ethnic background, sexual orientation or ability to qualify for or pay for such services.

Again, as Hospice Volunteer, You will start and continue on an endless learning curve. This will include coming to understand more about the Agency operation itself, the roles and ideals of Hospice within your community, your individual activities and responsibilities and how to interact with each newly assigned Patient.

BRIEF HISTORY OF HOSPICE TRADITIONS

Every culture has inevitably had to cope with the aging and dying of its members. There have been innumerable responses and perspectives on this universal Human experience across time. The exact historical origins of the ideals and practices of Hospice Care in western cultures are obscure. The first recorded references may be about the Knights

Hospitallers of St. John of Jerusalem. This quasi-religious military organization set up roadside inns to care for weary and sick travelers to and from the Holy Land starting during the 11th century Crusades. These Knights and their institutions were well established enough to be formally recognized by the Catholic Pope in 1113 as a distinct order. Some researchers have suggested that the modern concept of Hospice is thought to be derived from the Latin word *hospitium* which translates into hospitality or lodging. It also seems to be connected to the French word *hospes* which means host.

There is then little reference to something like Hospice care over subsequent centuries until the recorded work of St. Vincent de Paul who founded the Sisters of Charity in Paris, France in the 17th century. From that point forward, the unique practices of care designed specifically for people suffering an incurable disease spread through France, England, Ireland and Australia. Hospice traditions were brought to the United States in 1899 with the opening of the St. Rose Hospice by the Servants for Relief of Incurable Cancer. In these early pioneering institutions, care was generally provided through church funds and operated and staffed by religious monks and nuns, as well as lay volunteers.

Then, in 1905 the Irish Religious Sisters of Charity opened the St. Joseph Hospice in London. *Dame Cicely Saunders*, who is generally regarded as the founder of the modern Hospice movement, began her long career at St. Joseph's. Saunders was unique in that she brought her professional skills as a Nurse, Social Worker and finally a Physician to her Hospice work. She is credited with formalizing many of the noble ideals of the traditional religious orders in their compassionate care of the sick and dying, into more modern and scientific approaches. Then in 1967, she opened St. Christopher's Hospice outside of London, England. This was an innovative and revolutionary new facility dedicated exclusively to the Total Care of Individuals with a Terminal Disease, as well as their Loved Ones. It integrated the lofty aims of religious practice with the very best of modern Medicine and Psychology. St. Christopher's continues today as a worldwide leader in Hospice and Palliative care, education, research and advocacy.

Starting in 1963, Dame Saunders visited the United States to give a series of lectures on the Hospice movement in England. The American *Florence Wald* who was Dean of the Yale School of Nursing became a strong proponent of the approach. She organized Hospice, Inc. which eventually became the first modern Hospice facility in 1974 in New Haven, Connecticut. From that critical juncture, the number of Hospice facilities in the United States grew rapidly.

Then in 1982 the United States Congress passed a temporary bill expanding the national Medicare and Medi-caid systems to cover Hospice benefits. (Medi-caid is a medical Insurance system for low income people. It is operated as joint system funded by both federal and individual state resources). Organizations and Agencies who qualified with Medicare and Medi-caid could then be reimbursed for providing Hospice services within their communities. The Hospice Benefit provided under the umbrella of Medicare and Medi-caid was made permanent in 1986.

The National Hospice Organization was founded in 1978 and by 1980 had 138 member facilities. It has evolved into the National Hospice and Palliative Care Organization (NHPCO). As of 2015, there are over 6,100 agency locations offering Hospice services in the United Sates.

CHAPTER 2

PALLIATIVE CARE

▲ ▲ ▲

As a Hospice Volunteer, You may or may not be involved with a so-called specialized alternative to regular Hospice Care known as "Palliative Care". This will depend upon the policies and practices of the Agency You work with. Some Agencies offer "Palliative Care" support as an alternative to their more mainstream "Hospice Care" Program. These two approaches, Hospice and Palliative Care, share many common ideals and perspectives. However, there are some basic and practical variations between the two. These include differences in definitions and objectives, general settings within which they are offered, and ways in which they are managed and paid for.

In historical terms, "palliation" is a relatively modern development. The term *"Palliative Care"* was first coined by a physician named Dr. Balfour Mount around 1964 while working in Quebec, Canada. It is taken from the Latin word *"palliare"* whose root means "to cloak", as in to cloak or protect one from harm. Dr. Balfour's original intentions were to borrow the ideals within the growing Hospice movement and integrate them into a more general medical environment.

The American Academy of Hospice and Palliative Medicine states that the term "Palliative Care" has evolved over time. It originally referred to the care of individuals suffering with a terminal disease, but has now been expanded to encompass care designed for Individuals with serious chronic, life-limiting conditions. Such Care is no longer limited to Individuals that are imminently or actively dying.

Palliative Care programs encompass the following principles.

* The Palliative Care option can be chosen for someone facing a terminal disease or for one coping with a long-term severe chronic illness.
* Like Hospice, the overall objective is to maintain or enhance the highest possible Quality-of-Life for the Individual for as long as possible.
* Similar to Hospice, the Palliative approach seeks to engage the total Human Person, including physical, emotional, social, spiritual and existential issues.
* Unlike Hospice, Palliative Care does not require two Physicians to agree that the Patient has six months or less to live.
* The primary focus is on "comfort care", rather than "curative efforts". Palliation refers to the objective of mitigating or alleviating pain and suffering, without seeking to cure an underlying condition. However, endeavors to cure an ailment are never ruled out. If such an effort is deemed appropriate, treatment protocols can be subsequently pursued.
* Some specialized Hospice Agencies may offer a separate "Palliative Care" program within a private residence setting or Assisted Living Facility. However, the majority of Palliative support is delivered within a medical setting, such as a Skilled Nursing Facility (SNF), Sub-Acute Facility or an Acute Care Hospital.
* More and more hospitals are offering Palliative Care with regular hospital staff to care for Patients. Very few hospitals rely on outside Volunteer help within their Palliative Programs.
* Well over 90% of larger private and community hospitals now offer Palliative Care. Virtually all governmentally run hospitals, including every Veterans' Administration facility provide Palliative support.
* Palliative Care is not a separate Medicare, Medicaid or Medi-Cal Benefit. Instead, it is generally paid for as a regular Medicare benefit, or through regular private insurance benefits.

The medical component of Palliative Medicine earned formal status as a subspecialty in September 2006. With more and more Individuals eventually dying while in the care of a hospital facility, these institutions are providing Palliative support as an integral part of their overall healthcare programs.

CHAPTER 3

HOSPICE AND PALLIATIVE CARE FACTS

▲ ▲ ▲

HOSPICE CARE

THE FIRST FORMAL HOSPICE FACILITY in the United States was pioneered by Florence Wald in New Haven, Connecticut in 1974. During the years of 1982 to 1986, The U.S. Congress passed bills that authorized Medicare and Medicaid to reimburse qualified organizations for providing Hospice services. Over subsequent years Congress clarified the so-called "Conditions of Participation" (CoPs) for such qualification. These "conditions" required that unpaid Volunteers be a fundamental part of overall Hospice services. The Affordable Care Act (ACA) transferred the authorization of Hospice reimbursement from the U.S. Congress to the federal Secretary of Health and Human Services.

Each of these factors have fostered an explosive growth in the number of Hospice Programs currently operating in the United States. The following facts and numbers give a snapshot of Hospice care by 2015. (Source: NHPCO)

* There are approximately 6,100 "Programs" in the United States. This includes both corporate primary locations as well as satellite offices.
* Hospice programs are operated in a variety of settings. These include free-standing agencies-59.1%; as an integral part of a hospital system-19.6%; as part of a home health agency-16.3%; as part of a Skilled Nursing Facility-5.0%.

* The financial organizations of Hospice agencies take three formats: for-profit corporations-68%; not-for-profit agencies-28%; governmental agencies-4%.
* Payment for all Hospice services are provided primarily by three sources. Medicare-90.3%; Medicaid (Medi-Cal)-4.3%; Private Insurance-4.0%.
* Over 1.6 million Individuals receive formal Hospice care annually. This number increases each year.
* Over 1.2 million Individuals die while receiving some form of Hospice support. This number likewise increases each year.
* The most meaningful statistic for measuring the duration of Hospice service is the "median length of service" (LOS). This was 17.4 days in 2014. This refers to the so-called "50th percentile" which pinpoints the "median" quantity for how long Hospice services are provided. 50% of Individuals receiving Hospice care lived less than 17.4 days, while 50% lived longer than 17.4 days. (As distinguished from the "average length of service" which was 72.6 days in 2014. This takes into account the so-called statistical "outliers" that tend to distort the final calculation).
* Over 35% of Individuals opting for Hospice Support die in 7 days or less.
* Slightly over 10% of Individuals receiving Hospice Care survive longer than 180 days.
* Approximately, 84% of Hospice Care Recipients are 65 years or older.
* Ideally, Hospice care is offered within wherever Individuals reside. Those living in the Individuals' primary residence, including a private home, Assisted Living Facility or Skilled Nursing Facility-58.9%; In an Inpatient Hospice Facility-31.8%; In an Acute Care Hospital-9.3%.
* The Primary diagnoses for those receiving Hospice care varies widely. The largest proportion remains various Cancers-36.6%;

Various Dementias including Alzheimer's Disease-14.8%; Heart Disease-14.7%; Lung Disease-9.3%; Miscellaneous "Others"-12.9%; Stroke-6.4%; Kidney Disease-3.0%; Liver Disease-2.3%.

+ Again, t*here are approximately 430,000 Hospice Volunteers in the United States providing over 19 million hours of service annually.*

Palliative Care

Palliative Care Programs have likewise expanded tremendously in the United States in recent years. However, statistical data regarding such programs has not been compiled to the degree that data for Hospice programs have. Such information has been compiled for example, by the National Palliative Care Research Center (NPCRC). Numerical statistics have been calculated from information provided by hospitals and academic medical centers on an annualized "voluntary" basis.

For the most part, in the United states, Palliative Care programs have been developed as an integral part of the overall healthcare services offered within Acute Care Hospitals. As such, they utilize specially trained regular staff to provide care. In other words, such programs do not generally rely on outside Volunteer help, though there are always some exceptions.

Nonetheless, the following facts about Palliative Care can be identified within the year of 2015.

+ According to the National Palliative Care Registry, there are 683 hospitals reporting to offer formal Palliative Care programs within their facilities.
+ 67% of hospitals with 50 or more beds offer Palliative Care programs to Patients. This means that approximately 33% of such hospitals in the United States currently have no Palliative services.
+ Over 90% of hospitals with over 300 beds offer Palliative Care, while 56% of hospitals with less than 300 beds offer such a program.

- Virtually every governmentally operated hospital facility offers Palliative Care. This includes all the Veterans' Administration hospitals.
- Also, virtually every major Academic Medical Center offers a Palliative Care program.
- Not-for-Profit and public hospitals are four to eight times more likely to offer Palliative Care than are for-profit hospital chains.
- The "regional" prevalence of Palliative Care programs varies widely among geographical sections of the country. The highest percentage of hospitals offering Palliative Care is found in New England with 88%. In the west coast and Pacific region, it is 77%, while in the Mid-Atlantic it is 76%. The lower penetration for Palliative Care is found in west south central region at 43% and the southcentral area of the country at 42%.
- Medicare reports that approximately 78% of Medicare recipients who died in a hospital received Palliative Care.

Again, there are many similarities between Hospice Care and Palliative Care. They both endeavor to ease the Human burden during a tumultuous and desperate time. They both strive to promote the Quality-of-Life for Individuals suffering with severe disease or a life-threatening illness. Both try to address the total Human Person in this venture, as well as surrounding Loved Ones. The primary differences between the two approaches deal with variations in delivery logistics. These encompass the varying settings within which compassionate care is delivered, exactly who the team of professionals are that deliver that care and the methods through which such care is paid for.

Hospice and Palliative Care in American Society

▲ ▲ ▲

"Human Beings as well as healthcare professionals are so very often confused by the medical and existential questions of exactly when "living begins to end" and "dying begins to occur."

COL

"The most powerful and meaningful measure of a Human Life is the effect that Life has on other Human Lives."

Anonymous

"The best way to find yourself is to lose yourself in the service to others."

Mahatma Gandhi

WILLIAM

▲ ▲ ▲

OVER THE PHONE, THE VOLUNTEER Coordinator at Vitas asked me if I was a "sport fan" of any kind. I replied that "yes, I was a huge sports nut and a big fan of many different sports". She then asked me if I would be willing to take on a new assignment that included a very specific request. The Patient's name was William and he had been active in sports during most of his life as a player, coach and referee. He was now 86 years old and had been suffering with Parkinson's Disease for over 28 years. It was evident to the attending Doctors that William's life was now drawing to an end. He was continuing to live within his private home cared for by regular Hospice staff and his devoted wife and sons. An electric hospital bed had been placed in his bedroom facing a large screen television.

The family had agreed to have a Volunteer pay periodic visits "if that Volunteer could and would discuss various sports topics" with William. He was very restricted in his ability to verbalize conversation, so the Volunteer would have to be able to carry on the lion's share of the inter-action. This was a perfect assignment for me as I was a man, a big talker and a sport fan.

As a Volunteer, I would pay a visit to William's bedside about once a week. I always prepared for my visit by reviewing all the major sports stories going on at the time. I would be ready to review college and pro-fessional players, performances, records, schedules, standings, etc. on all the active sports. Again, as William could only strain to form a few simple questions or comments, I would talk for the majority of the time we spent together. If there was a daytime game on, we would watch that on the television and I would offer a running commentary on the action. As with all Hospice visitations, I always tried to be keenly aware of William's energy and comfort levels. The actual length of each visit was determined by how I perceived William was feeling. Sometimes they lasted only 45 minutes and at other times they would last up to an hour and a half long.

My visits with William lasted about six weeks. Then I was told by the Agency that he had declined significantly and that I should probably wait to try to see him again. Then within a couple of weeks, I was informed that William had passed peacefully in his home surrounded by his Family. My assignment was over.

CHAPTER 4

END-OF-LIFE ISSUES

▲ ▲ ▲

OVER RECENT DECADES, THERE HAVE been multiple "Psychosocial Surveys" conducted asking elderly People what they think about dying and death. If they have lived long enough, they have usually witnessed the decline and disease and eventual death of Friends and Loved Ones. They have also experienced their own gradual internal physical and cognitive loss of vitality and acuity. They are usually grappling with multiple chronic conditions. While enduring these natural and inevitable patterns of Human Life, they have reported some very powerful and insightful observations on these subjects. Three of the most striking are these.

1. The vast majority of Elders are not actually afraid of "being dead". They may not like the idea in the long run. But, generally speaking, older Individuals have each sorted out their own belief systems about the pervasive questions of life after death, heaven, the soul, oblivion and what they might expect with "no longer being alive". However, what these Surveys do reveal is that older People are very much afraid of the "process of dying". They fear the inherent unpredictability of this final stage. They fear the "possible" pain and confusion, the gradual incapacity, the loss of simple functional abilities, the loss of personal control, the loss of work and activities, the loss of cognitive abilities, the loss of relationships, the loss of any joy and the ultimate loss of the Human Self. They almost unanimously express the terrible

fear of becoming a burden to others. They dread the prospect that such things might drag on for many months or even years. Again, it is the frightening uncertainty of not knowing exactly how such a process might play out.

2. These Surveys also report the so-called "80-20 Rule". The vast majority of Seniors (80%) claim that at the very end of their lives, they would prefer to die in their own "home setting" surrounded by close Loved Ones. This means that a much smaller number of Elders (20%) say they would prefer to die within a fully supported professional medicalized environment. The harsh reality is that the actual facts about mortality in the United Sates turn out to be almost exactly opposite to these stated wishes. Fully 80% of Americans end up dying within some sort of medical "facility", such as an ambulance, an emergency room, an ICU, a hospital, sub-acute facility, skilled nursing facility, or even an assisted living facility (which is sometimes regarded as a "home setting"). Only 18-20% of older People die at home in relative peace with close Loved Ones in attendance.

3. Still other Surveys reveal a very curious sentiment among older People. A large majority of these Individuals (75%) state that if given the option, they would prefer to die in their sleep. Again, this reflects a generalized fear or anxiety about consciously facing the final end of the "process of dying".

It is precisely these kinds of deep and far-reaching Human attitudes that the traditions and ideals of Hospice and Palliative Care seek to address. These programs are designed to lessen or ameliorate the frightening perspectives and experiences that these Surveys reveal about the Human encounter with dying and death.

1. Hospice and Palliative Care strives to maintain or enhance the current physical, emotional, spiritual and social well-being of both

Patient and Loved Ones. Signs and symptoms of pain and distress are dealt with directly. Personal hands-on support is provided to help compensate for functional losses or cognitive declines. In Hospice, whenever possible, Patients are kept in their home-setting, with Loved Ones being trained on and providing much of the daily care. Patients and Family receive spiritual support and counseling as requested. They are also provided with on-going professional assessments of what may be transpiring in terms of the diseases and what might be expected. Professionals have termed this kind of support "anticipatory understanding" of the process of dying and death. Grief and Bereavement support and counseling are offered both before and after the death of the Patient.

2. As mentioned above, the Hospice approach endeavors to maintain Patients within their chosen "home setting" as much as possible. This serves as an attempt to achieve the personal wishes revealed in the "80-20% Rule. People prefer to die at home with Loved Ones. A common pattern is for some Patients being cared for by the Palliative Care Team within an acute care hospital to be subsequently transferred back into their "home setting" where continuing care is taken over by a Hospice Agency.

3. It is a curious but basic medical reality that most Individuals who die within Hospice or Palliative support die while asleep or unconscious. They usually pass quietly and peacefully. They have often endured a complex and difficult long-term disease trajectory. In terms of effective pain and symptom management, they have often received increasing levels of pain medication and have been prescribed sedatives to relieve distress. Towards the very end, they often sleep a great deal and go in and out of consciousness. Dying is sometimes so quiet as to be almost imperceptible. Breathing is often drawn out and erratic and then simply stops. So, the 75% who prefer to die asleep usually get their wish.

DYING AND DEATH IN CONTEMPORARY SOCIETY

There is nothing so daunting to Human Beings as being forced to confront their own mortality, or that of a close Loved One. This entails nothing less than grappling with the inevitable recognition that all life is fragile and ultimately transitory. Every life form on this planet will ultimately disintegrate and pass away. Human Beings have great difficulty with the prospects of their own extinction, as well as that of the Individuals with which they love and share their lives. People usually endeavor to avoid the so-called "Grim Reaper", either through the auspices of traditional religious appeals and rituals or through modern medical interventions. The generic biological instinct to survive at all costs manifests in Humans as the all-encompassing "will to live". In the overall course of a Human Life, the single greatest challenge and tragedy Individuals face is usually the death and final loss of a Loved One. The grieving Survivors are never really quite the same after such a profound and intimate loss.

The astounding advancements in modern medicine and technology have had a massive impact on how modern Americans live and die. As mentioned before, life expectancy in 1900 was around 47 years in the United States. Now it is pushing past 80 years of age. On average, Individuals are living longer, as well as being healthy and active longer. It is now commonplace for an Individual to be totally cured from a serious disease that often proved fatal a few short decades ago. That Person then survives for many years, only to subsequently be struck down by a still more lethal disease that ultimately takes the Person's life. Paradoxically, as a result, People now are generally sicker and debilitated longer with an array of chronic conditions that emerge with a longer life. Still, it remains a biological fact that Individuals mature and grow old very differently. While a few People remain vital, mentally sharp and physically active into their 90s, others become incapacitated in their 50s or 60s. The Human reality of the "process of growing old" has become enormously complex and unpredictable in the United States.

Likewise, as revealed in the three survey themes above, the American experience of dying and death has become increasingly complex and confusing. When an Individual contracts a serious illness, that Patient may well be cured and recover to a fully healthy life. In other cases that illness may progress and cascade into multiple life-threatening conditions (co-morbidities) and finally death. Different Individuals with seemingly similar conditions and identical medical diagnoses may go through very different experiences. When such similar Individuals consent to and undergo identical treatment protocols, the medical outcomes can vary widely. For example, roughly 50% of Adults receiving bone marrow transplants for various leukemias are free of the disease five years later. This means 50% are not. The unsettling fact is that no one knows with absolute certainty how a serious disease will progress nor what the outcomes of a specific approach to treatment will be until "after" the disease and treatment have run their course. In the complex arena of illness and treatment strategies, each individual Human is unique. What consists of "medical futility" for one Person may turn out to be a "miraculous cure" for another Person. This is why medical Professionals express treatment "outcomes" in terms of demographics, percentages and time frames. (e.g.- "Evidence based statistical analysis shows that 68% of Individuals with similar demographics and identical diagnoses who receive this specific treatment protocol are free of the disease 5 years later. This also of course means that 32% had very different outcomes").

Modern medicine has undergone another fundamental evolution over the past few decades in the United States. Prior to this cultural shift, disease treatment options and decisions were generally left in the hands of Physicians. However, in recent times, "Patient-Centered" Care and decisions are now assigned to the Patient whenever feasible. The Physician's role is ideally to elaborate various treatment options including potential benefits and associated risks. The Physician is usually asked to make specific recommendations concerning treatment options and outcomes. Thereafter, the Patient makes medical choices based on the information provided. An adult Patient cannot "demand" any specific medical treatment without a Physician's agreement. However, a Patient may choose among various treatment options offered and that Patient also has the right to "refuse" any and all medical treatment protocols. As a reflection of this cultural evolution, the "Patient Self-Determination Act" passed by the US Congress in 1998 requires all government-funded Health Providers to give Patients the opportunity to formally articulate their ideals and preferences for End-of-Life treatments when admitted to a Medical Facility.

It is no wonder that Americans are generally not well prepared when they or any Loved Ones are struck with a life-threatening condition. Exactly how a Person or a Loved One will respond to treatments designed to cure a serious illness is uncertain. In general, People hope that modern technology and advanced medical strategies will produce a cure. In many cases, they do. In others, they do not. The strict distinction between living and dying has become terribly blurred in modern America. Again, Individuals Patients as well as healthcare professionals are so very often confused by the medical and existential questions of exactly when "living begins to end" and "dying begins to occur".

With the extraordinary successes of modern medicine to thwart the ravages of serious diseases, it is not surprising that People try to utilize any and all relevant medical strategies to save Themselves or a sick Loved One. When suddenly faced with a life-threatening condition, many People often voice their resolve to "never quit", "never give up", "leave no stone unturned", "spare no expense", "never ever give in" to that illness. This is a natural reflection of the personal biological will to live, or to the deep and desperate affection and attachment to Loved Ones.

THE HOSPICE AND PALLIATIVE CARE OPTION

Yet, inevitably Human Beings perish. Modern technology and cutting edge medical advancements have found no absolute cure for dying and death. In every single battle against mortality, Human Beings ultimately lose. The challenging question for Patients and Loved Ones becomes at what point during serious disease and gradual decline does "comfort care" become the most viable option. When does Hospice or Palliative support become the very best strategy for the overall Quality-of-Life of a Person suffering with a life-threatening condition for the reminder of that Individual's lifetime? Arriving at such a conclusion is always the end result of a long and arduous and tumultuous journey for both the sick Patient and concerned Loved Ones. There are often vehement disagreements within the immediate Family about finally taking this course of action. In certain instances, the Patient may express a desire to pursue no further invasive treatments, while Family Members may desperately want to continue such efforts. In many more extreme situations, the Patient may be suffering some degree of cognitive decline, in which case the process of decision making becomes that much more confusing and difficult.

Medical personnel also play a critical role in the complicated process of choosing the Hospice or Palliative Care option for an Individual Patient. This is a difficult arena for which many Physicians and Nurses are not well prepared. Their education and training and on-going efforts are all directed towards healing and defeating serious diseases. Finally choosing and recommending only "comfort care" going forward may seem to connote professional failure. At this critical juncture, the medical battle against illness has been effectively lost. All their best treatment strategies have been in vain. Now, they have to "deliver bad news" to Patients that have put a lofty trust in them and their acumen at healing. Yet, the role of Physicians is central to the decision to opt for Hospice or Palliative support. It is they who must clearly affirm that there seems to be "nothing further that can be done in terms of curing the disease". Their careful analysis and explanation of the Patient's condition is crucial to how that Patient and close Family Members think about the decisions at hand. However, the overriding principle that "should" guide this rarified decision is that ultimately the personal wishes of the informed Patient must be respected and carried out as much as possible.

Finally consenting to the Hospice or Palliative Care option generally encompasses several critical turning points in thinking and attitudes on the part of the Patient and hopefully close Family Members. The option does encompass an emotional coming to terms with the biological reality that all things pass away and that includes "myself" or "my dying Loved One". (see Kubler-Ross's five stages to gain a sense of just how difficult this is). This includes a fundamental resignation to the idea that the disease or diseases are essentially unassailable and ultimately incurable (again, a strategic assumption in Palliative Care is that further treatments at curing may be considered at some point in the future). Choosing the Hospice or Palliative option also implies that further aggressive, invasive and often painful treatment protocols are not only considered futile, but that they may cause further severe physical and mental suffering. In other words, they will have no meaningful effect on the course of the disease and may well diminish the Patient's Quality-of-Life for whatever time remains.

Once the critical decision has finally been made to defer to the Hospice or Palliative Care approach, several key issues become paramount. Researchers in a very revealing study concluded in 1999 had asked terminally ill Patients what they wanted most over the remaining course of their lives. Five primary themes emerged.

1. *" to avoid becoming a burden on Family and Loved Ones".*
2. *"to maintain a sense of autonomy and control".*
3. *"to have physical pain and other distressing symptoms managed effectively".*
4. *"to focus on and enhance personal relationships as much as possible"*
5. *"to avoid futile or inappropriate prolonging of the underlying dying process".*

Again, similar to the three Psychosocial Surveys above, the core ideals and "Best Practices" within the Hospice and Palliative approaches strive to address each of these challenging issues for Individuals struggling with a life-limiting disease. Whether a Patient is currently maintained in a hospital or in a home setting or anywhere else, they are supported by a multidimensional team of Caregivers. Physicians, Nurses, Social Workers, Aides, Counselors, Therapists, Volunteers, etc. all endeavor to ease the daily burdens of both the Patient and Loved Ones. This is designed to lessen the Patient's anxiety of being too big of a burden to Family Members.

At every step along the process, the Patient's personal wishes are protected and respected as much as possible by the team of Caregivers. From the very start of Hospice or Palliative Care, special attention is given to Patient autonomy in the form of medical and financial "Advanced Directives" as integral parts of care strategies. It is sometimes helpful for Patients and Loved Ones to understand that at any given point in time, they are free to opt out of Hospice or Palliative Care. They are under no obligations to continue in these systems once they have started. So, if a Patient somehow stabilizes, regains strength and even shows signs of a recovery, they can return to a regular medical treatment regime at any time. On-going counseling and discussions are a part of the daily routine and changing circumstances.

Effective "symptom and pain control" is central to Hospice and Palliative Care. This entails the on-going management of physical pain as well as mental, emotional, spiritual or existential anxiety and distress. Again, these factors are addressed by the various members of the "Interdisciplinary Team" of active Caregivers. As the Patient's condition and circumstances change so does the practical hands-on prescriptions and care.

Another central tenet in Hospice and Palliative support is the encouragement and engagement with surrounding Family Members and close Friends in the care and decision making about the Patient's overall well-being. The personal relationships of the Patient with various People always take on a renewed power and meaning. Connections and reconnections with important Persons take on a profound importance. Sometimes even estranged relationships with certain People are rekindled.

When pressed for an answer, most People will state that they do not want any extraordinary medical procedures to be performed if and when those procedures will ultimately fail. This is especially true among older Individuals concerning invasive treatments that may cause further pain and suffering and offer no prospects for success. There is the realization of the intrinsic value of focusing on Life and Family and enjoyable activities for as long as possible. This is often more appealing than an endless series of oppressive trips to the emergency room or days spent in the sterile medicalized environment of the ICU in order to survive a few more days or weeks. Again, in seeking to respect the Patient's inherent right to determine the decisions and course of their dying and death, Hospice and Palliative support endeavors to carry out these private wishes as much as possible. Again, each of the above five profoundly intense sentiments are directly addressed within the auspices of both Hospice and Palliative Care approaches. They are too often ignored or overlooked in the normal course of medical testing, diagnosis, assessing a prognosis and curative treatments designed to achieve healing, at any cost.

IN SUMMARY

Inevitably, all life forms on this exquisite planet pass away. As difficult as this is to accept, this includes "me" as well as "my Loved Ones". Coming to terms with the reality that "I" will someday perish is difficult for most to cope with. Witnessing the dying of those dear to "me" is usually the hardest Human experience "I" will endure.

The extraordinary advancements in medical science have extended the American life expectancy dramatically over recent decades. This has emerged as a demographic "two-edged sword". People are now routinely living into their 80s and 90s. While they are often healthy and active longer, they are also then incapacitated longer with a litany of chronic diseases. Many of these conditions are associated with simply living longer lives. Ultimately, seven of the ten leading causes of death in People over 65 years of age are attributable to complications caused by chronic illnesses. The actual course of these ailments is usually complex, and unpredictable. They develop over many years and fluctuate in symptoms and severity.

For these reasons, it has become more and more difficult to evaluate End-of-Life issues. It has become exceedingly problematic to determine when "living ends and dying begins" for any specific Individual. As medical and pharmaceutical achievements continue, it will become still more challenging to deal with these Human factors in the future.

And yet again, all Human Beings perish without exception. The desperate question remains about how to best navigate these complicated situations. Hospice and Palliative Care stand as one very powerful and meaningful course of action in response to a Person's inexorable physical and mental decline. At some point, the critical and pivotal decision may be made by the Patient, supported by Loved Ones and sanctioned by medical professionals to opt for "comfort care". In this case, an entirely new set of priorities and perspectives are adopted. Generally, a new set of Professionals and Caregivers springs into action and the Patient's daily routine changes. The primary objective becomes exclusively the Quality-of-Life for the Individual on a day-to-day basis for whatever time remains.

In historical terms, Hospice and Palliative Care have only recently become formally integrated within the American healthcare systems. Hospice was finally approved as a permanent Medicare benefit in 1986. It took individual states longer to dovetail Medicaid benefits to reflect federal certification. Palliative Care was finally sanctioned and recognized as a medical specialty in 2006. Yet, there is still an inherent resistance to the admonition to opt for Hospice and Palliative Care within American society. Human Beings resist dying. Loved Ones resist giving up. Medical professional resist quitting.

However, the approach and ideals of Hospice and Palliative Care have emerged as a hallmark of Human caring and dignity and reverence for the sanctity of Human life during the most difficult of all Human experiences. No doubt, its powerful role as an integral part of a compassionate and effective healthcare system will only expand as time goes on.

CHAPTER 5

HUMAN AGING OVER THE LIFECOURSE
DISEASE – DYING - DEATH

▲ ▲ ▲

DEFINITION: *"LIFE COURSE"* DESCRIBES AN Individual's passage through an entire lifetime. It analyzes a Human life as a series of significant "stages" and pivotal "events". These encompass biological, cultural and social dimensions. This includes such issues as age, heredity, health, education, marriage, work, religion, old age and death. This approach endeavors to understand the Whole Person over an entire life as lived.

When working as a Hospice Volunteer, it can be enormously helpful to have a basic understanding of how Human Beings live, grow, decline, develop life-threatening conditions and eventually die. Although You will quickly begin to realize that every single Individual's experience that You work with is utterly unique, there are general biological patterns that Human organisms tend to follow over the Life Course. If You are aware of these patterns, it will be easier for You to engage the People You spend time with in a meaningful way, even in the midst of their difficult and tumultuous journey.

In general, most of the Patients You will be working with will be at an advanced age. You will be spending most of your time with Hospice in the company of elderly people. The primary reason for this is simply that as People grow older, they become more susceptible to various diseases. As Individuals pass through middle age and beyond, they tend to develop a range of "chronic illnesses" which can become life-threatening over time. For this reason, it will be beneficial if You have a clear sense of what being elderly is like.

AGING OVER THE LIFE COURSE

The Human Species generally follows a basic biological pattern over the so-called "Life Course". The vast majority of People are born relatively helpless, they develop and mature and grow in terms of energy, vitality and capacity. They become stronger and more able to engage life and its' challenges. Then, they tend to "plateau" physically and cognitively in their 20s and 30s. Thereafter, Individuals begin to slowly decline in terms of power and effectiveness. This slowing down occurs within a molecular, cellular, organ, systems and overall physical prowess level. This inevitable decline occurs at very different rates among different People. Yet, this is the natural course of virtually all biological forms.   Simply growing old does not mean that something has gone wrong or that the Individual is suffering with a "disease".

However, it is the case that as Humans grow more elderly, they are less capable of warding off or fighting various diseases. As their physical strength and energy wanes, they become more susceptible to illness. Among other issues, an older Person's immune system becomes less capable of resisting disease. Also, older Individuals endure more years of accumulated environmental and lifestyle stress and effects.

Commensurate with this natural life cycle is the fact that the Human Mind also grows strong and capable, then plateaus and then tends to decline in acuity and capacity. A 25 year old tends to be better able to listen, learn, comprehend, retain and analyze new information than an 85 year old. Again, this does not mean that something has gone wrong with the older person. As the physical body declines, so does the Human Mind.

One of the most respected and best known studies of Human Aging is the Baltimore Longitudinal Study of Aging (BLSA - sponsored by the National Institute on Aging – a division of the National Institutes of Health). This on-going study identified 24 specific physiological "Biomarkers" that were used to assess the long-term biological and cognitive changes associated with Human aging over many decades. These include such factors as blood pressure, sensory acuity, kidney efficiency, sugar regulation and uptake, immune response to environmental stressors, etc. Starting in 1958 and continuing in the present, while surveying as many as 3,100 individuals, the overall data and conclusions were uniformly clear. While Individuals age very differently, virtually every one of the 24 Biomarkers revealed a decline in efficiency associated with increasing age. All Humans follow a generic pattern of biological, cognitive and functional growth, plateau and gradual decline.

Individual Human Beings age very differently. Some people remain healthy and active into their 90s, while others are incapacitated by the age of 50. Besides genetic makeup and lifestyle patterns, social and economic factors can weigh heavily on the way in which Individuals grow old. The Centers for Disease Control (CDC) reports that the average surviving 75 year old American suffers with three chronic illnesses and takes five prescription medications.

The Human patterns and experiences of disease, debility and death have undergone a fundamental cultural shift in American society. In previous centuries and well into the 20th century, most deaths were caused by infectious diseases, childbirth and accidents. Death was very common in infancy, childhood and young adulthood. Dying was usually quick and unanticipated. In 1900, the average "life expectancy" in the United States was around 47 years of age. Now at the start of the 21st century, it is around 80 years. Many common diseases or infections or life-threatening accidents are now routinely treated, eliminated or cured.

This remarkable situation is the long-term result of many complex factors. These include improvements in sanitation and personal hygiene, ready access to abundant food and nutritional resources, emergency medical response systems, preventative and diagnostic medical advancements and a vast array of high-tech surgery and treatment pro-tocols. Enormous advances in pharmaceutical technologies have had a huge effect on medical efficacy. The development of antibiotics, ste-roids, high-blood pressure medications, statin drugs, insulin manage-ment systems, chemotherapies for cancer treatments, blood thinners, pain medications, etc. have reshaped the course of Human disease, de-bility and mortality. Likewise, anti-psychotics, anti-depressives, and anti-anxiety medications have improved the daily Quality-of-Life for millions of Americans.

Again, the accumulative effect of these unprecedented advancements is that Americans are now living longer than ever before. The average age of Individuals in the United States is increasing. This is sometimes referred to as the "graying" of America. The fastest growing segment of the population on a percentage basis is the so-called "Oldest-Old". These include those 85 years and older. In the year 2010 there were 40.2 million Americans 65 and older in the United States. In 2030 this num-ber will increase to 71.5 million. By the year 2050, the population of the United States will include 86.7 million Seniors.

This explosive growth in the number of Seniors is also due largely to the impact of the "Baby Boomer Generation". This refers to the huge upswing in the number of births between the years of 1946 and 1964. This so-called "bulge" in the aging demographic includes over 77 mil-lion people. The first wave of the Baby Boomers started to turn 65 in 2011. Now, every day on average, over 10,000 of these Individuals join the ranks of Senior Citizens. This staggering trend will continue for 19 years. That is 10,000 per day, 70,000 per week and 300,000 per month for 19 years.

But, these extraordinary achievements have fostered an inherent par-adox. The reality is that while Individuals are living longer and longer, they are also then subsequently sicker and debilitated longer. This also reflects the fact that People are generally healthy and active longer than their parents and grandparents. Also, for many the actual dying pro-cess is often artificially extended through medical interventions. Modern medicine has developed the extraordinary capacity to prolong life, even in the face of progressive and inevitable aging.

The extraordinary achievements in modern medicine have actually had a profound effect on how Americans think about disease and treatments and the expectations for a cure. People have been conditioned to look to hi-tech medical interventions to remedy even the most intractable diseases and conditions. Modern medical science has been naturally buoyed by its long litany of dramatic cutting-edge breakthroughs and healing successes. All these and many more have fostered a deep and pervasive cultural assumption that Human diseases can be thwarted and life can be extended again and again.

ACUTE AND CHRONIC DISEASE

Modern medicine generally divides diseases into "acute" or "chronic" categories. The strict medical distinction between acute diseases and chronic diseases is often arbitrary and can even change over time. *"Acute diseases"* usually have specific identifiable causes, such as an accident or bacterial or viral infections. They often have an abrupt onset and may be completely cured within a relatively short timeframe. They usually include symptoms and often physical distress and pain. Examples of acute diseases can include pneumonia, flu, measles, mumps, strep, stroke and certain advanced cancers.

"Chronic diseases" can be loosely defined as "degenerative health problems" that persist over an extended period of time. Chronic diseases are generally non-contagious, have a long latency period, and they fluctuate in severity and the duration of symptoms. They usually manifest slowly and get progressively worse over time. They are often regarded as irreversible and ultimately incurable. Once developed, they often continue throughout a Person's remaining lifetime. Another long-term consequence of the increase in chronic conditions is that seven of the top ten leading causes of death in the United States are now attributable to the complications caused by various chronic diseases.

Some chronic conditions are mild in effect, some are debilitating and some are life threatening. These ailments and their complications are the leading reason why Seniors visit their doctors. They are the primary reasons for the majority of emergency room and hospital visits. Managing chronic diseases are why 1.5 million Residents are living permanently in the nation's nursing homes. They are the major causes of long-term disabilities. As they progress, they have an increasingly limiting effect on Elders' daily activities, emotional well-being and social engagements. Ultimately, they often cascade eventually to death, directly or indirectly.

Nowadays, most Individuals who live for many years gradually end up struggling with a variety of long-term "chronic conditions or diseases". It is one of the unintended consequences of extending the length of Human life. Circumstantially, many Americans now simply live long enough to contract a variety of chronic diseases. It is difficult, if not impossible to differentiate between a predetermined genetic course of aging and the ongoing impact of environmental and lifestyle choices. Again, as People grow older, they tend to become more susceptible to disease. Their biological capacity to first resist contracting disease diminishes. Likewise, their ability to fight disease once contracted also lessened. As mentioned, in spite of these facts, growing elderly in itself is not a disease. The process of growing old does not mean that something has gone wrong. Like infancy, puberty and young adulthood, being elderly is a natural part of the overall Life Course.

In medical terms, the most meaningful course of treatments for chronic conditions are designed to simply manage the "signs and symptoms" and daily impact on the Individual's Quality-of-Life. Examples of chronic diseases can include asthma, bronchitis, diabetes, high-blood pressure, osteoporosis, arthritis, Parkinson's disease, kidney failure, congestive heart failure, progressive dementias and certain cancers.

It is sometimes difficult for senior citizens to recognize the distinction between "normal aging" and the onset of various chronic illnesses. Many elders end up living for many years with multiple chronic conditions. Many eventually die from those same conditions. There is often a blurring of the dividing lines among growing older, the onset of a multitude of chronic conditions, the development of serious and acute illness and final mortality. In modern American society the distinction between when "living ends" and "dying begins" has become increasingly impossible to specify.

In terms of medical economic issues, perhaps most striking of all is that fully 75% of all medical expenditures in the United States go to treat chronic illnesses. That is three of every four dollars spent. Also, virtually 95% of all expenditures for Seniors are spent to manage chronic conditions and their consequences.

Researchers have developed an array of "Theories" to describe and explain Human Aging over the Life Course. These include Psychological Perspectives such as *"Stages of Personality Theory"*, *"Life Course Theory"*, *"Selective Optimization Theory"*. Sociological approaches include *"Continuity Theory"*, *"Gerotranscendence Theory"* and *"Age Stratification Theory"*. Biological frameworks include *"Free Radical Theory"*, *"Wear and Tear Theory"* and *"Programmed Genetic Theory"*. The most basic fact is that Aging is an enormously complex process and can be approached in a multitude of ways. Yet, every single Human Person is subject to it. To be Human is to age, to grow elderly and to eventually die.

VOLUNTEER PREPARATION

▲ ▲ ▲

"Our personal anguish, grief, confusion, anger or sense of injustice over watching the death of a cherished Loved One is ultimately the Human cost we pay for loving others; that in the myriad course of Human things, if we live long enough and love others deeply enough we will inevitably suffer sorrow and grief."

COL

People may well forget exactly what You said or what You did, but They will never forget how You made Them feel!"

M. ANGELOU

"No act of kindness, no matter how small is ever wasted."

AESOP

Fred and Carmen

▲ ▲ ▲

I FIRST MET FRED AND his wife Carmen in August of 2009 at their modest suburban home in Daly City, California. In-home Hospice Care was being provided to the couple by Pathways Home Health and Hospice out of the South San Francisco office. Fred had been diagnosed with terminal throat cancer and was spending his days and nights resting in a powered hospital bed strategically placed in the living room. He was effectively bed-ridden at all times. He had a permanent tracheostomy to allow for breathing. He also had a feeding tube inserted into his stomach for nutritional and drug delivery. He also had a catheter for easy voiding of urine. He had daily visits from the Agency Home Health Aide to perform regular care. The Agency Nurse visited three to four times each week. Also, Carmen had been trained by the Agency staff to perform routine around-the-clock care of Fred.

My modest role as a Hospice Volunteer was simply to visit once a week to allow Carmen some "respite" time away from her very demanding situation. She would leave the house to run various errands. She might pick up groceries, go to the bank, pick up dry cleaning, go to the post office or visit friends. She would usually be gone about two hours. I was always struck by how calm and kind and appreciative she appeared to be when I was there. I assumed this reflected a strong and courageous character. When she returned she would always thank me profusely with a big smile and a warm hug.

Whenever I first arrived, I would shake Fred's hand while he reclined upright in the raised bed. He always seemed to recognize me and would give me a warm and sincere smile. I never heard his voice, as by that time the cancer and medical interventions had robbed him of the ability to speak. Carmen would usually administer a liquid dose of Ativan (an anti-anxiety drug) into his feeding tube to help keep him calm during her absence. When she left I would sit next to Fred's bed and we would watch his favorite TV shows which included several court room dramas such as Judge Joe Brown and Peoples' Court. Once in a while, I would comment about the shows and he would acknowledge me with his eyes. In general, very little was said. Sometimes in these situations mere words seemed intrusive and jarring. During my visits, Fred would sometimes sleep for most of the time.

I visited Fred and Carmen weekly for just over four months. During that time, Fred's health conditions slowly declined. He became progressively less animated and would sleep more and more. Then at my last visit, Carmen seemed especially warm and attentive and said how much they appreciated my visits. But, she went on to explain that their daughter was going to be moving back into their home and would be there to help with the daily household routine and challenges. They had decided as a family that this would be best for the remaining time. So, she thanked me over and over again and said that they would no longer need my visits. I thanked them for the opportunity to share in their journey. I was subsequently informed by Pathways that Fred had died about five weeks after my last visit. As always, I sent a personal sympathy card expressing my appreciation to the family for letting me be a small part of their lives.

CHAPTER 6

GETTING STARTED

▲ ▲ ▲

ASSUMING THAT YOU HAVE MADE the decision to offer your time and effort as a Hospice Volunteer, the steps to be taken are fairly simple. The practical fact is that Hospice Agencies are always engaged in efforts to recruit new Volunteers. They are in fact compelled by Medicare Regulations to maintain on-going activities designed to promote Volunteer resources and training within their organization and the communities they serve. If You are a sincere, compassionate and willing Person they will usually be open to discussing Volunteer opportunities with them.

You may already know of one or more Hospice Agencies in your area. You may have already interacted with various Hospice personnel caring for a Family Member or close Loved One. You may have Friends who have received Hospice Support for a Loved One. You may have come across an educational speech or public forum where Hospice Support was being promoted within the community. If You live in or near a town or city of any size, there should be a Hospice Agency near You. Again, there are over 6,100 locations that offer Hospice Support in the United States.

Of course, You can always find specific Hospice Agencies near You on the internet. On the computer, You can research individual Agencies and get some feel for their size and approach and history. The next logical step is to contact the Agency and ask to speak to the "Volunteer Coordinator". You might discuss various questions that You have over the phone, or You can schedule an initial appointment to meet the Coordinator. Sooner or later they will want to meet You in Person.

Keep in mind that for legal and regulatory reasons, You as a Volunteer are considered to be an "Employee" of the Agency and must comply with all relevant policies and procedures. So, if You and the Agency come to a mutual decision to proceed, they will generally require several basic steps be followed before formal Training begins. These include the following.

* Application
* Personal References
* Personal Background Check
* Tuberculosis Test
* Basic "Employee" Physical

Some Agencies may stipulate additional requirements such as the following.

* Flu Shot
* MMR (Measles-Mumps-Rubella) immunity. A prospective Volunteer may satisfy this requirement by producing a current "vaccination record". You may also demonstrate valid immunity through the presence of MMR "titers" that are present through a clinical blood draw. If neither of these factors are available, You may submit to new vaccinations. (MMR immunity is not required by federal regulations, but certain Hospice Agencies do choose to require it of their Volunteers)
* Fingerprinting
* DMV Record, Certification of Automobile Registration and Insurance if your car will be used in any form of Volunteer activities.

Hospice Agencies generally have regularly scheduled Training sessions set up during the course of a calendar year. For example, they may have formal Training classes that begin in the spring and then again in the fall. You will generally be scheduled to participate in one of these sessions. These classes are designed to help You learn about the philosophy and traditions of Hospice Care, the practical operations and obligations of the Agency and your duties and responsibilities as a Volunteer.

Initial Volunteer Training

As a Hospice Volunteer, your formal involvement will begin with a focused and highly structured series of classes. This vital Training is required by the Agency itself, as well as Federal and State Regulations. Proper Volunteer Training is likewise stipulated by Medicare and Medicaid for Agencies seeking certification for financial reimbursement for Hospice services. If You are new to Hospice, this introduction to the field will be invaluable. You will meet with your Volunteer Coordinator, various members of the Interdisciplinary Team, seasoned veterans working in the field, as well as other new Volunteers like yourself. You will be exposed to the general history, philosophy and ideals advocated by Hospice traditions. You will also be introduced to the specific policies, procedures and programs maintained by your Agency within this complex field.

The exact scope and agenda of this initial training will vary among different Agencies across the country. This variation is acceptable within the purview of Federal Statutes. The Code of Federal Regulations stipulates that:

> *"Standard Training. The Hospice must maintain, document, and provide volunteer orientation and training that is consistent with hospice industry standards".*

These very generalized requirements allow a great deal of practical leeway for individual Agencies to develop different approaches to Training Programs. As a new Volunteer, You should simply absorb whatever itinerary and topics your Agency offers. Keep in mind that they are the seasoned experts, they know what they are doing and they are sanctioned and certified by both State and Federal regulatory bodies. You will be learning from Individuals who have worked for many years in this challenging field.

The actual length of hours of your initial Training may also vary among Agencies. In the past most introductory Programs for Hospice extended to 30-40 hours of Training. Nowadays, with People having such busy schedules, most Agencies require approximately 20-25 hours of focused Training covering a "core curriculum" of themes. These sessions will often be conducted over a couple of weekend classes or over a series of weeknight classes. Agencies will routinely offer introductory Training at certain regular intervals during a calendar year. Once You have committed to working as a Volunteer, contact your Agency to find out when their Training classes are scheduled. If their regular Training is not for some time, they may be able to offer a provisional Training Program wherein You meet with individual staff members and even "tag-along" with more experienced Volunteers.

Different Agencies will utilize different training methods and materials with their new Volunteers. These may include lectures, guest speakers, panel discussions, group exercises, writing exercises, videos, take home assignments and written tests. You will also receive a Training Manual covering everything you cover during the introduction as well as many other related subjects. It is suggested strongly that You read through this material thoroughly, as it will explain in detail many issues not adequately covered in your 20-25 hours of classwork.

The following is a summary of specific themes that are generally covered in all introductions to Hospice.

- *Introduction to the Agency:* This is usually a brief overview of the organization's origins, history, management structures, locations and geographical areas served and range of services offered.
- *History and Development of Hospice:* This encompasses a brief survey of the cultural roots and evolution of Hospice traditions in the West. It details the explosive growth of Hospice Agencies over recent decades in the United States.

- *Survey of Hospice Ideals:* This describes the approach and objectives of Hospice within contemporary society. Hospice endeavors to offer a more compassionate approach to these final journeys than the more medicalized environment of the emergency room or the hospital. Ideally, Family and Loved Ones are trained and supported as the essential "unit-of-care" in the Patient's routine care.

- *Explanation of the Interdisciplinary Team or Group:* This details the specific members of the Care Team, including their various roles and responsibilities in the approach to total Patient support. Volunteers learn that they are regarded as an integral part of this close-knit team. Their direct contact and experiences with Patients is invaluable to the Team's on-going assessment of that Patient.

- *Volunteer Communication Channels:* This includes the primary Agency Staff Members to which the Volunteer will routinely report. This also explains the Staff Member the Volunteer will call in the event of a significant problem or emergency during a visit. This would obviously include if the Patient actually died during a solitary visit.

- *Explanation of various types of Volunteer Activity:* This outlines the many types of roles Volunteers may engage in working with the Agency. This includes Friendly Visitor, Respite, Vigil, Transportation, Grief and Bereavement Support, Clerical work, Phone Work, Event Support, Fund Raising as well as many others. The Agency will strive to match new Volunteers with the areas of service they prefer to work in.

- *Communication Skills:* This concerns the highly sensitive arena of interacting with Patients struggling with a life-threatening disease, as well as surrounding Loved Ones. Volunteers are guided in specialized abilities such as empathetic listening, nonjudgmental conversation and nonverbal communication.

- *Overview of Dying and Death:* This delves into the experiences of dying in contemporary society. This generally includes descriptions of the complex changes in the physical, emotional and cognitive conditions and behaviors of a dying Patient. Special emphasis is given regarding the types of diseases Hospice Patients commonly suffer with. Volunteers are given some insights into the "signs and symptoms" they may encounter when dealing with Patients.

* *Social Network Dynamics:* This is designed for the Volunteer to develop some sense of the complexity and the intensity of what a dying Patient's Family and Loved Ones also endure. Everyone is suffering a profound and desperate loss. This can cause tremendous stress on the Social Network around the Patient. It is critical for the Volunteer to be cognizant of these issues.

* *Grief and Bereavement Services:* This outlines the specialized form of compassionate care offered to surrounding Family and Loved Ones who also endured the dying and death of the Patient. All Agencies certified by Medicare are required to provide a full 12 months of Grief and Bereavement support following the death of the Hospice Patient. Volunteers interested in this line of work will undergo an extra course of training and involvement with staff.

* *Patients' Rights and Confidentiality:* This deals with the responsibility of the Agency to inform both the Patient and close Loved Ones of certain procedural guidelines. These include fundamental principles such as Respect and Dignity, Patient Autonomy and Confidentiality. As an integral member of the Hospice Care Team, the Volunteer will be required to abide by these important rules and procedures at all times.

* *Record Keeping and Activity Reports:* This details the routine personal logs and Activity Report Forms the Volunteer will need to turn into the Agency. The Agency is required to maintain these reports on file and will regularly use the information provided as part of the on-going Care Plan and assessment of the Patient.

* *Self-Care:* This explains the importance of Volunteers being aware of their own cognitive, emotional and physical health while

carrying out their duties with Hospice. Volunteers are directly engaged with Human Beings who are often sad, exhausted, frightened, angry, confused, depressed and grieving. This can have a profound but subtle impact on the Volunteer. It is paramount for Hospice Volunteers to develop strategies to maintain personnel well-being.

* *Specialized Volunteer Activities:* This will be a brief survey of the various other forms of Volunteer roles that might be considered. These may include a Pet Visit Program, Spiritual or Religious Counseling, Massage, Reiki, Arts and Crafts, Cosmetology, Phone Check-Ins, Music and Entertainment, Events and Fund Raising, Public Speaker and Community Liaison for Hospice, Thrift Shop Staff as well as a variety of Clerical Support Positions. These specialized activities will require the Volunteer to undergo extra training and working with various Staff Members.

Following completion of the initial Hospice Training Program, You will generally meet privately with the Volunteer Coordinator. This may be immediately following the final class or it may be scheduled at a later date. During this important meeting, You can openly discuss any issues or concerns or questions that might have come up about the Training or your role as a Hospice Volunteer. Even though you are considered an integral part of the Interdisciplinary Team, your primary connection and interaction with the agency will be through the Volunteer Coordinator. You should always feel that You can be completely honest and forthright with this Person. The Coordinator will always be highly supportive of You, your experience and personal welfare.

During this follow-up interview, You will discuss the specific Volunteer assignments that may be available to You and which assignments You prefer to pursue. Keep in mind that the most common Hospice Volunteer assignments will be as a Friendly Visitor. These may include assignments in a variety of settings, such as a Private Residence or an Assisted Living Facility. The conditions of the Patients and the circumstances of Family and Loved Ones will vary tremendously. Each assignment is unique. You may well walk out of this first meeting with your coordinator with an initial assignment, or You may have to wait for some time thereafter to get this first Volunteer opportunity.

If this is your very first Hospice work, the Agency will generally require that a seasoned Volunteer go with You on your initial assignment. Depending on how quickly You develop confidence during your visits, this experienced Co-Volunteer may go on several of these visitations with You. This Person can take the lead and allow you to observe the interactions with the Patient and any Loved Ones present. This is the so-called "on the job training" so valuable to new Volunteers. Following your visits, You can ask your fellow Volunteer any questions that have occurred to You in the course of the visit. This seasoned Volunteer may be able to make observations and offer suggestions to help You. You may want to discuss your initial visits with your Coordinator. Your Agency is keenly interested in guiding your experiences and supporting your efforts during the early stages of your involvement.

The following chapters describe several key topics in more depth. As You progress in your activities as a Volunteer, You will become increasingly aware of how these issues support and guide the policies and procedures of the Hospice Agency in End-of-Life care.

CHAPTER 7

THE INTERDISCIPLINARY TEAM --
INTERDISCIPLINARY GROUP

▲ ▲ ▲

DURING YOUR INITIAL TRAINING, YOU will be introduced to the concept that, as a Hospice Volunteer, You are regarded within the Agency as an integral part of the "Interdisciplinary Team" (IDT) Team or "Interdisciplinary Group" (IDG). This Team or Group of Individuals are those within the Agency that are directly responsible for the initial and on-going care of the Hospice Patient and surrounding Loved Ones. Federal Regulations stipulate that all certified Hospice Agencies maintain effective Patient support in the areas of "Physicians Services", "Nursing Services", "Social Services" and "Counseling Services". Minimally, this Team or Group must include a Doctor of Medicine (MD) or Osteopathy DO), a Registered Nurse, a Licensed Social Worker and a Licensed Counselor. Together these Professionals are mandated to provide care and support for the Total Human Patient, including the *physical, psychological, social, spiritual and existential dimensions* of the Person, as well as Family and Loved Ones.

However, within the practical organization of the Hospice Agency, the IDT or IDG consists of a team of a much wider range of Individuals with specific skill-sets and responsibilities. Although there will be some variation among Agencies, the typical team or group will usually include the following positions.

* _Medical Director:_ This MD or DO will have the responsibilities to oversee the clinical and administrative policies and practices of the operation. This Doctor reviews incoming cases and certifies whether Patients qualify for Hospice services as well as subsequent re-certification as appropriate. The Director is generally available for medical consultations and will work with members of the IDT/IDG as needed. This Individual often serves as a representative and advocate for the Hospice approach to End-of-Life Care within the wider medical community. This Doctor may assume primary responsibilities for a Hospice Patient, if that Patient's regular Physician prefers to turn such care over to a medical professional that is more experienced in terminal situations.

* _Primary Care / Attending Physician:_ This is usually the regular or long-term Doctor that has followed the Patient for years. This is often the Physician that refers the Patient to Hospice Care when all conventional treatment efforts to cure a serious disease have been exhausted. This Doctor is always a critical source of medical information and experience with the Patient. This Physician may or may not continue to serve as the Primary Care Physician for the Patient while under a formal Hospice Program. As mentioned, this Professional will often voluntarily turn control of medical decisions and prescriptions over to the Hospice Medical Director.

* _Registered Nurses (RNs):_ Each Agency will have a variety of specific nursing roles and responsibilities within the organization. They will serve as an initial Assessment Nurse for in-coming Patients and as an on-going Case Manager. As such, they are actively engaged in the development and monitoring of the Patient's individual Care-Plan. Field Nurses will routinely visit Patients and surrounding Loved Ones within their home setting to evaluate their current conditions and circumstances. Visiting Nurses will carefully guide and instruct Family Caregivers in proper handling and administration of daily care, including managing Activities of Daily Living (ADLs), medications and any on-site medical equipment. They

will provide emotional support and help Patients and Family to understand what to expect as the underlying disease progresses and as the final end draws near. Nurses serve as the pivotal liaison and advocate between the Patient and Family and the Interdisciplinary Team.

* *Nurse's Aides:* These Individuals are usually trained as Certified Nurses Assistants (CNAs) or specifically as Home Health Aides (HHAs). These field workers are truly the unsung heroes in Hospice Care in that they provide the lion-share of daily direct hands-on care to the Patient within a private residence. They perform a variety of duties that are difficult for some Family Members and yet do not require a Registered Nurse to accomplish. These might include cleaning or bathing, shaving, brushing teeth, feeding, transferring to a wheelchair, doing nails, hair, makeup, etc. Because of their on-going daily interactions with the Patient and surrounding Caregivers, they are often the closest and most trusted members of the entire Hospice Staff. Patients and Family Members sometimes confide a great deal in them. Therefore, the Nurse's Aide's judgements and observations are often very important to the Agency IDT and the evaluation of the Patient's Care Plan.

* *Licensed Social Worker (LSW):* These are specialists in the social and logistical issues surrounding End-of-Life Care. The Hospice Social Worker will assist with the initial Assessment of new Patients and the development of a Care Plan tailored to that Person. The LSW will seek to understand the changing psychosocial dimensions of the Patient and surrounding social network. This Person may be called on to help the Family navigate through personal conflicts and difficulties. The Social Worker will introduce information concerning Advanced Directives about Financial and Medical autonomy, authority and decision making. Without giving legal advice, The LSW may explain the strategic importance of Wills and Trusts and Estate Planning in End-of-Life situations. The Social Worker will likewise enlist the support of various community and

governmental resources when appropriate for the Patient and Family. If necessary, the LSW can assist with the mortuary, funeral and any memorial services planned by the Family.

* _Counselor_: Virtually every single member of the IDT that interacts directly with the Patient and Loved Ones can serve as a supportive Counselor in some capacity. However, within most Hospice Agencies, there are two types of Counselors that may be utilized for specialized contributions. The first of these is the professional Licensed Psychologist or even Licensed Psychiatrist who may be called upon for formal therapeutic guidance. These professionals may be kept on a legal retainer or act of independent contractors. The second type of Counselor that may be used is the Spiritual Counselor. This Person will specialize in religious or theological perspectives concerning the Human ordeals of sickness, suffering and death.

* _Volunteer Coordinator_: This individual serves as a pivotal liaison between the overall organization of the Hospice Agency and the pool of various Volunteers working both in the field and the central office. As such, the Volunteer Coordinator oversees all aspects of Volunteer activities. This includes on-going recruiting of new Volunteers while promoting the message and ideals of Hospice Care within the community. It entails conducting preliminary interviews of prospective Volunteers. It encompasses all phases of initial Training and follow-up Training. It includes managing all mandated screening and testing of Volunteers, such as Criminal Background Checks, TB tests, physical exams, valid identifications, driver's license, etc. It requires that all relevant records and current information about Volunteers be updated and kept on file. The Volunteer Coordinator attends all IDT meetings to review on-going issues regarding Patients. This includes initial Assessment evaluations to develop a strategic Plan of Care for each Individual. The Coordinator oversees and implements all incoming and on-going Volunteer assignments. This can be

a daunting challenge as many larger Agencies will often have 200-300 Patients at any one time. The Coordinator is required to enforce compliance with all Medicare, Medicaid and Corporate regulations concerning Hospice Volunteer activities. For example, each Agency is required to maintain activity logs and be able to demonstrate the "5% Rule", requiring that fully 5% or more of all "direct hands-on care" of Patients be provided by unpaid Volunteers. The Coordinator is required to train and demonstrate Volunteer competence in such areas as "HIPAA", and state Safety Laws. The Volunteer Coordinator and the supporting Staff within the Volunteer Department truly have a massive and complex job.

* *Grief and Bereavement Coordinator:* Medicare Regulations require that all certified Hospice Agencies provide Grief and Bereavement Care to any and all Loved Ones following the death of the Hospice Patient. This specialized support must be available for at least 12 months after the death. The Bereavement Coordinator or Director is responsible for all aspects of these services. Such activities might include periodic phone calls to Family Members. It may include scheduling personal one-on-one visitations with specially trained Bereavement Volunteers. It usually entails implementing and managing various Grief and Bereavement Support Groups within the community. The Coordinator may refer bereaved Family Members to Professional Therapists in cases of "complicated grief". The practical reality is that most Hospice Agencies will offer Grief and Bereavement support to the community at large, not only to Families who had a Loved One under formal Hospice Care.

In addition to the "Core Members" of the IDT or IGT described above, there are a variety of other skilled Professionals and trained Individuals who may play a critical role with Hospice Patients in certain situations. In keeping with the essential Hospice Approach to End-of-Life Care, each of these Caregivers bring support designed to maintain or enhance the temporary physical or emotional "comfort" of the Patient. Each of these types of services requires some form of specialized training or education or certification. Some of these activities are routinely provided by Volunteers while others may be offered by paid Professionals. Such extra caregiving services might include *Physical Therapy (PT), Occupational Therapy (OT), Speech Therapy (ST), Massage Therapy, Acupuncture, Acupuncture, Aromatherapy, Pet Therapy, Reiki, Meditation*, etc. Obviously, the range of such extra support services varies widely from one Hospice Agency to another.

DISCUSSION OF VOLUNTEER ISSUES

Again, Medicare Regulations require that unpaid Hospice Volunteers be an integral part of the Interdisciplinary Team. As such, Volunteers are called upon to provide a minimum of 5% of all direct hands-on Care of Patients. Certified Agencies must be able to record and document this level of participation by Volunteers. As a Hospice Volunteer, it is helpful for You to recognize the importance your Coordinator will put into implementing and maintaining your Volunteer activities with Patients. It may take some time for You to get used to the fact that You are considered a vital Member of the IDT /IDG.

The IDT / IDG Members have regularly scheduled Meetings to review the conditions, changes or issues concerning Patients being served by the Hospice Agency. Your Hospice Coordinator will usually attend these general Meetings to report the activities and experiences of Volunteers in the field. The Coordinator serves as your advocate and representative during these important Meetings. The vital information and feedback You as a Volunteer in the field provide the Coordinator becomes part of the on-going assessments of Patients. Your Activity Logs and all other input becomes a permanent part of the Patient's Case File.

It is important for You as a Volunteer to develop a clear understanding of your significance to the IDT / IDG. Your importance may not be readily apparent because You usually perform your duties in the field, outside the physical offices of the Agency itself. You usually do not rub shoulders with the Agency Staff on a regular basis. Once You are trained and confident, many or most of your interactions with the Agency and the Coordinator will be through the mail, over the phone or the computer. You may go for weeks or even months without stepping foot inside the Agency offices. Nonetheless, You are always thought of as a vital part of the Team.

As a Hospice Volunteer, You are always welcome to attend regular IDT / IDG Meetings that assess any Patients You are currently visiting. In fact, the Coordinator will always encourage You to do so. You should attend at least several of these Meetings during your early work with the Agency. It is highly suggested that You do this in order for You to develop a wider sense of the roles and interactions of Team Members and your specific place there.

As a fundamental part of the IDT / IDG, You should always feel free to connect with other Members of the Team to discuss issues surrounding the Patients You are visiting. You can generally do this over the phone or through emails (as governed by relevant HIPAA policies). You will routinely interact with the Coordinator about significant changes or problems with Patients. However, at certain points it may be beneficial for You to speak directly to the visiting Nurse or the Social Worker or the Spiritual Counselor about specific topics. Examples of such issues that You may have observed could be a dramatic change or decline in functional or cognitive status. The general consensus within the Agency is that the more "eyes and ears" that interact with each Patient, the more meaningful the Care being provided. This is why your interactions and observations with individual Patients are so valuable.

It is very important for You as a Hospice Volunteer to keep in mind just how hectic and busy most Agency Staff are during the workday. The Volunteer Coordinator and department Staff often oversee the Volunteer support of dozens or even hundreds of Hospice Patients. These Patients' prognoses and conditions are often in a state of enormous complexity and fluctuations. The Coordinator is responsible for all Volunteer promotions, training, field assignments, record keeping, regulatory compliance, etc. within the Agency. Likewise, Case Managers, Visiting Nurses, Home Health Aides, Social Workers, Counselors and Bereavement Coordinators are usually enormously busy with responsibilities for many Patients. It is important for You as a Volunteer to be mindful and respectful of Team Members when You do interact with them and they with You. Teamwork is the foundation for an efficient and effective Agency.

CHAPTER 8

MEDICARE – MEDICAID
HOSPICE FEDERAL AND STATE REGULATIONS

▲ ▲ ▲

MEDICARE

Medicare is a National Healthcare Insurance Payment System. It is regulated, administered and funded by the US Federal Government. It was first enacted by Congress in 1966 during the Johnson Administration. It is designed to provide Healthcare Insurance protection for American citizens 65 years and older. It also provides Healthcare support to all younger Persons who are collecting disabilities benefits under Social Security Disabilities Insurance. These Medicare benefits are offered to Individuals regardless of personal income or medical conditions. Medicare is currently managed by the Centers for Medicare and Medicaid Services (CMS) which is an integral component within the Department of Health and Human Services. With the first members of the "Baby Boomer Generation" turning 65 in 2011, the projected cost to provide Medicare benefits in the year 2022 will exceed $1 trillion annually.

Over the years Federal Medicare Regulations have undergone several major revisions. In the watershed year of 1982, an initial temporary provision for Hospice funding was drafted as part of the Tax Equity and Fiscal Responsibility Act. Hospice Care was funded and made available on a temporary trial basis in 1983. Then in 1986, the Medicare "Hospice Benefit" was made permanent as a specialized provision within Part A of the Medicare Program. The basic Federal Medicare Hospice Regulations are found in Title 42 – Part 418 *("42CFR418") of the Federal Code.* Over the following years, there have been a series of expansions to the Federal Regulations as "Interpretive Guidelines" issued to clarify the "Conditions of Participation" (CoP) required for independent Hospice Agencies to qualify for Medicare reimbursement.

From the very beginning of the expansion of Medicare benefits to include payments for Hospice services, Volunteers have been an integral part of any qualified Agencies daily activities. This regulatory requirement was put into effect to both save operating costs and to honor the long historical traditional ideals of Volunteers caring for the most desperate of terminally ill People.

The specific provisions of the Federal Code concerning Volunteers within a Hospice Agency are fairly simple and succinct. They encompass the following key points.

- The Hospice Agency must use Volunteers to a minimum extent in defined roles and under the direct supervision of a designated employee.
- The Agency must provide, maintain and document Hospice orientation and Training consistent with industry standards.
- Volunteers must be utilized in daily administrative or direct Patient Care activities.
- The Agency must demonstrate and document viable and on-going efforts to recruit and retain Volunteers.
- The Agency must calculate, document and record the actual "cost savings" achieved through the active utilization of Volunteers.
- The Agency must require that Volunteers provide administrative or direct Patient Care that is equivalent to a minimum of 5% of the total Patient Care hours provided by paid and contract employees.

The practical reality is that these very brief Regulations allow a tremendous leeway in exactly how individual Hospice Agencies use Volunteers in their day-to-day operations.

MEDICAID

Medicaid is a Healthcare Insurance Payment System that is administered and funded jointly between the Federal Government and Individual States. As such, it is managed by both the Centers for Medicare & Medicaid Services (CMS) and individual State Agencies. Medicaid is designed to offer benefits to low-income and no-income Individuals regardless of health status.

In 1986, Individual States were given the option by the Federal Government to include a Hospice Benefit within their individual Medicaid Programs. In concert with the development of Hospice Insurance Benefits on the federal level, most states gradually refined their own Medicaid Hospice Programs following 1986 to better serve low-income People in their own states. Though there are some minor differences among the various states concerning the policies and procedures of delivering Hospice Care, the basic Programs are very similar. For specific provisions within any state, the individual State Medicaid Agencies should be consulted.

MEDICARE – MEDICAID HOSPICE BENEFITS

Certified Hospice Agencies receiving payments through either the Medicare or Medicaid Programs must be capable of providing the basic Services listed below.

* Physician Services
* Nursing Care and Support
* Home Health Aide Care
* Social Work Support
* Psychosocial Counseling
* Grief and Bereavement Counseling
* Physical Therapy
* Occupational Therapy
* Speech Therapy

- Dietary Counseling
- Appropriate Medications
- Medical Supplies
- Medical Equipment
- Short-Term "In-Patient" Care for severe symptom management or Respite support.
- Short-Term "at-home" continuous Care during periods of extraordinary crises.

This does not mean that all Hospice Patients will routinely receive all of these benefits. Every Patient's situation is unique and the Agency's Interdisciplinary Team will develop and monitor an individualized Plan of Care for each Person. In addition to those listed above, other Hospice Services may include any specialized care and treatments deemed "medically necessary" by a following Physician to provide the best "comfort care" possible for the Patient.

MEDICARE ELECTION AND CERTIFICATION OF HOSPICE BENEFITS

Federal Regulations stipulate that Hospice Benefits will be provided initially through two successive periods of 90 days and thereafter for an unlimited number of 60 day periods as necessary. The approval for each new period requires two Physicians to certify that the Patient is not expected to live longer than six months assuming the underlying disease runs its expected course. So, the initial 90 days benefit period requires the two Physician certification and each subsequent benefit period requires recertification by two Physicians. The benefit periods within individual States' Medicaid Programs vary somewhat. Again, each States' Regulations should be consulted.

The practical medical reality is that it is exceedingly difficult to predict the course and time-line of a life-threatening disease. It is almost impossible to pinpoint the actual time of death before it happens. Every

Hospice Patient's experience is unique. This is why Federal and State Regulations governing Hospice Benefits require certification and then recertification by two Physicians engaged with the Patient for each benefit period. It is also why Hospice Benefits can and will be provided indefinitely if necessary, during an open-ended series of 60 days benefit periods.

Hospice Benefits are an "elected benefit" provided for in Medicare Part A. When a Patient chooses to enroll in Hospice, that Person no longer receives general medical coverage under Part A. The terms and conditions for Hospice healthcare support are tailored to the unique circumstances of a Patient coping with a life-shortening illness. Federal Regulations require that a Person choosing to enroll in Hospice do so voluntarily, within the medical guidelines of "informed consent". In cases of significant functional or cognitive problems, a duly assigned Representative or "Medical Proxy" can choose Hospice Care for an impaired Patient.

Likewise, a Patient or legal Representative can choose to stop active Hospice Care at any time. This falls within the purview of "Patient's Rights" both according to Federal and State Regulations, as well as all Hospice Agencies. For those Individuals under Medicare and Medicaid who opt out of Hospice Care, they will automatically resume support under the regular provisions of those Programs.

MEDICARE HOSPICE LEVELS OF CARE AND REIMBURSEMENT

Federal Medicare Regulations specify four basic "Levels of Care" for Hospice support of Patients. Each Level deals with varying degrees of activity and support. Each of these Levels is reimbursed at a different "per diem" or daily flat rate. These include the following.

1. *Routine Home Care (RHC):* This usually includes visits by an RN several times a week and often a Home Health Aide on a daily basis. Social Services and Counseling are available upon request.

As of January 1, 2016, this Level of Care will be reimbursed at an accelerated rate higher for the first 60 days of services and at a subsequent lower rate thereafter.

2. *Continuous Home Care:* This entails some form of intensive and continuous on-sight presence of Agency Caregivers. This is usually offered during times of heightened difficulties or crises.

3. *Inpatient Respite Care:* This usually includes the situation wherein a Hospice Patient is actually placed in a facility of some kind in order to provide Family and Loved Ones with a "respite break" from the intensity of personal hands-on home care.

4. *General Inpatient Care:* This deals with the extreme situation wherein a Patient simply cannot be properly taken care of in the "home setting".

With the implementation of the Affordable Care Act, there have been several modifications to the reimbursement structure for participating Hospice Agencies. One of the most significant is the "Service Intensity Add-on" payment (SIA). This essentially increases the amount of payments for services rendered during the final 7 days of a Patient's life. This is in recognition of the practical fact that often during this critical period, the required level of engagement and care services increases dramatically.

Another important change to Medicare's overseeing Hospice care is the adoption of the so-called Hospice Quality Reporting Program (HQRP). This is a relatively new attempt to assess the actual Quality of Care administered by Agencies as delivered to Patients. The program is still undergoing basic implementation and evolution.

The scope and principles of Medicare regulations of Hospice Care are becoming more and more complex. Ideally, this increasing complexity will make the Quality of Patient Care, as well as the fairness of payments for services rendered more effective and efficient. Hospice Care is a continuously improving sector of the American Healthcare system.

CHAPTER 9

HEALTH INSURANCE PORTABILITY AND ACCOUNTABILITY ACT (HIPAA)

▲ ▲ ▲

MODERN MEDICAL PRACTICE HAS UNDERGONE a fundamental evolution over the past few decades in the United States. Prior to this gradual cultural shift, disease treatment options and decisions were generally left in the hands of Physicians. However, in recent times, "Patient-Centered" care and decisions are now assigned to the Patient whenever feasible. The Physician's role is to arrive at an accurate diagnosis of a disease and to then elaborate various treatment options. This includes the potential benefits and associated risks of such treatments. The Physician is generally asked to make specific recommendations concerning these treatment options and outcomes. Thereafter, the Patient ideally makes medical choices based on the information provided. Within this modern medical environment, an adult Patient cannot "demand" any specific formal treatment without a Physician's consent. However, a Patient may choose among various Treatment options offered and that Patient is also afforded the right to "refuse" any and all medical treatment protocols. These factors can become significant in End-of-Life situations.

As a consequence of this "Patient-Centered" approach to medical care, one of the most significant changes in modern medicine has been the recognition of the critical importance of "Patient Autonomy" and "Patient Confidentiality" within any and all medical settings and facilities. In response to this growing need, the United States Congress passed the *"Health Insurance Portability and Accountability Act"* in 1996. These regulatory guidelines are often referred to simply as *"HIPAA"*.

Essentially, this legislation was designed to assign exclusive control of a Patient's medical records to the Patient, or to a duly appointed Medical Proxy. A Patient's medical conditions and history are considered private and confidential and will only be shown to those Individuals to whom the Patient grants access. Such information is often referred to as *"PHI"* or Protected Health Information. This encompasses any facts or details that might identify a Patient within a public setting. This might include full name, address, social security number or a specific medical diagnosis.

Maintaining such protection and confidentiality can be tricky with the advent of the digital revolution. This has had a profound effect on the electronic transmission and sharing of Patient's private medical records. Such sharing may be between a private Physician's office, an Emergency Room, a Hospital, a Skilled Nursing Facility, an Insurance Carrier, etc. Each of these medical entities are held accountable for maintaining HIPAA Guidelines. Each is required to maintain Patient privacy. Each is called upon to obtain "Informed Consent" from the Patient to have access to medical information.

HIPAA regulations also apply to Hospice Agencies and Hospice Care. The personal confidentiality of Patients receiving Hospice support must be maintained at all times. This has a powerful structural impact on the daily operations of Hospice Agencies. This also requires some simple guidelines on how Hospice Volunteers interact with Patients and the Agency.

Generally, after a Volunteer has listened to a basic description of a potential assignment and has agreed to take that assignment on, the Agency will provide all important and relevant personal and medical details about the Patient. The Volunteer is free to ask any pertinent questions that may affect the Volunteer's interaction with the Patient and any surrounding Loved Ones. In essence, the Patient granted the Agency the right to share such information with an assigned Volunteer. This "Informed

Consent" was obtained during the initial "Admission Agreement" between the Patient or Medical Proxy and the Hospice Agency.

However, from the initial visit, the Volunteer needs to continue to maintain HIPAA guidelines in all aspects of Patient activities. If the Hospice Volunteer maintains private and confidential information within the home about the Patients that that Volunteer is seeing, strict rules apply. The Volunteer must keep all written or recorded information about a Patient in a "secure" location, such as a locked file cabinet. The Volunteer should not discuss any identifying details about a Patient with Friends or Family. Even when corresponding with the Hospice Agency, certain rigid guidelines must be maintained. Any specific identifying information about a Patient should never be included in a routine email. This is because emails are considered as potentially public information. So, when sending an email to the Volunteer Coordinator, the Volunteer may refer to a specific Patient by using that Patient's initials only. For example, *"Patient S.W. was alert and oriented during my visit on Tuesday"*. Those agencies that use computer platforms for Volunteers to forward "Activity Logs" will have their own password protection to maintain HIPAA principles.

Again, as always Hospice Volunteers will be trained thoroughly in HIPAA regulations during their Initial Training. HIPAA regulations will always be integrated into Volunteer activity. If any confusion or questions come up, the Volunteer should look to the Volunteer Coordinator for guidance. This will be a basic part of the steep learning curve each Volunteer undergoes as they expand Patient interactions.

CHAPTER 10

PATIENT "HOME" SETTINGS

▲ ▲ ▲

WITHIN A COMMUNITY, HOSPICE AGENCIES strive to offer their support services to any Individuals facing a life-threatening illness. The ideals and practices of Hospice are designed to maintain Patients in their chosen "home" setting for as long as possible, surrounded by their close Family and Loved Ones. This means that Hospice is active within a wide variety of "home" settings. Within this context, "home" encompasses wherever Patients are presently residing or regard as their residence. With Americans living longer than ever before, a Patient's "home" may be living in a "Private Residence", or spending the remainder of their lives in an "Assisted Living Facility" or a "Skilled Nursing Facility". Some Agencies have even reported working with Patients who are homeless or living temporarily in a public shelter.

The harsh reality is that People facing a life-limiting disease often spend their last days and weeks and months in a variety of support settings. This might include sudden visits to an acute-care hospital for emergencies, temporary rehabilitation in a nursing home, spending time with relatives for short-term care and eventually back to the Patient's primary residence. The specific current location will usually be dictated by the Patient's active medical conditions, cognitive status and functional abilities.

Wherever the Patient is dwelling, Hospice Volunteers will be called upon to travel there and offer their unique brand of compassionate care. To newer Volunteers, some of these complex settings and facilities may seem a bit intimidating. Hospitals and nursing homes are often a whirl-wind of many different personnel and activities through which a Volunteer may have difficulty navigating.

It is important for new Volunteers to have a basic understanding of the various types of settings they may be asked to visit. These include the following.

Private Residences: This encompasses any and all independent home dwellings where a Patient may reside. This can include a house, an apartment, a condominium, a private room within a community house, a long-term hotel room, etc. In unusual circumstances, a Patient may live alone for some time. It is far more common for a Patient to live with a Spouse or Partner. Often Patients may end up living with various other Family Members or close Loved Ones, such as with a Sibling, or Adult Children or Adult Grandchildren.

Assisted Living Facilities (ALF): This is by far the fastest growing part of the Elder care housing and support segment of the American society. These types of facilities are generally regulated on a state level only (there are no federal national regulations that oversee their routine operations). There are various licensing designations within each state for the vari-ous forms Assisted Living can take. These can range from independent living communities (as e.g. within California and other states, one type is the "Continuing Care Retirement Community" or "CCRC".). Assisted Living Facilities can encompass small single home dwelling care units, large complex locations supporting dozens or hundreds of Residents, and even large national for-profit corporations operating many facilities in multiple states. (Again, in California the umbrella licensing category for most Assisted Living Facilities is the "Resident Care Facility for the Elderly" or "RCFE"). Small home settings caring for six Persons or less are licensed as RCFEs and are often referred to as "Board and Care" units.

In general, Residents in an Assisted Living Facility enjoy a high degree of personal freedom and autonomy. They usually have a private dwelling that may be a single room or they may be in a multi-room apartment setting. They may live alone or with a Spouse or Partner. ALF Residents do not require continuous 24-hour nursing care. However, facilities do routinely offer a variety of progressive levels of support for their Residences, as needed. Individual "levels of care" programs can be tailored to each Individual or Couple. ALFs generally provide meals and housekeeping services to all. Beyond that facilities will offer assistance with various "Activities of Daily Living" (ADLs), such as dressing, feeding, toileting, transferring, etc. They will also offer assistance with medications and laundry. They will provide transportation to various locations outside the facility, such as church services or shopping destinations. They will generally have regular programs for activities and outings. They strive to provide a positive and stimulating and supportive home environment to all their Residences.

In general, financial support for living within ALFs are not provided for through Medicare. There are a few individual small Board and Cares which accept a limited number of Medicaid (in California – Medi-Cal) supported Residences. For the most part, living in an Assisted Living Facility must be paid for by private insurance or as a Family out-of-pocket expense.

Skilled Nursing Facility (SNF): These are generally "In-Patient" facilities for Individuals with illnesses or disabilities requiring 24-hour skilled nursing support. These facilities are tightly regulated by both Individual States and Federal Statues. As such they must adhere to strict State and Federal guidelines in order to qualify for financial reimbursement through Medicare and Medicaid, as well as through private insurance programs.

In large Skilled Nursing Facilities, there are usually two major sections segregating types of care. The first is the temporary or "rehabilitation" section. If Individuals have recently been in an Acute Care Hospital, they are often referred to a Skilled Nursing Facility for follow-up rehabilitation work. Typical forms of rehabilitation efforts may include Physical Therapy, Occupational Therapy or Speech Therapy. For example, a

Patient undergoing knee replacement surgery may be placed into a SNF to "rehab" from that procedure. The stay there is expected to be short-term or temporary. For Individuals who suffered a stroke, went to the hospital's emergency room, subsequent referral to a Skilled Nursing Facility for follow-up rehab is very common.

The other major Section within many SNF is the permanent, long-term care or "custodial care" ward. This includes Patients who continue to require 24-hour nursing care on a continual basis. This encompasses those who "live out their lives in a nursing home', as they are medically, cognitively or functionally unable to live in a private residence or in an Assisted Living Facility.

Rehabilitation care for Elders in a SNF is generally paid for by Medicare Part A. It is a limited reimbursement scale covering 20 days fully, then 80 more days with a required co-payment. In general, Medicare does not pay for long-term custodial care. The practical financial reality is that in most cases Individuals residing permanently in a SNF end up as Medicaid (or Medi-Cal) recipients. For many aging Seniors, this is the ultimate healthcare safety net after personal financial assets have been exhausted.

Memory / Dementia / Alzheimer's Care: Another specialized form of Elder care encompasses support for those suffering with various forms of debilitating "cognitive decline". As People are living longer and longer, these afflictions are becoming more and more prevalent within the American healthcare landscape. Medical science claims there are as many as 75 potential causes for cognitive problems. Some are mild and temporary, while others are progressive and irreversible. As People grow older, there is a natural and "normal" decline in mental sharpness and acuity. However, cognitive deficits can be serious and eventually fatal. The most common form of severe decline is Alzheimer's Disease, which is ultimately incurable and life-threatening. Other forms include vascular dementia, temporal-frontal lobe dementia, Lewy-bodies dementia.

Because of the increase of these diseases, so-called "Memory Care" or "Dementia Care" units have been developed within many Assisted Living Facilities as well as Skilled Nursing Facilities across the country. Such programs require conforming with very specific regulatory oversight. On a state level, ALFs must qualify for a "Dementia Waiver", while SNF must comply with both state and federal regulations. Within both settings, personnel staff must be trained and certified to work in this complex and challenging field.

As a Hospice Volunteer, You may be asked to visit a wide diversity of Patients within any of the locations described above. The more assignments You take on, the more comfortable and confident You will become.

WORKING WITH PATIENTS - LOVED ONES

▲ ▲ ▲

"It has been said that an Individual's life is best understood as a personal narrative of a series of 'stories'. To recount a Person's biography is to describe that life as a story. As with all Human Beings, that Person's private story intersects with Others' life stories and must be understood within the wider arena of still other social and cultural stories".

COL

"my being merely Human is hopefully what makes my presence here worthwhile. We can spend time together reminiscing, laughing, and crying. You can tell me about your youth, your family, school, work, interests, joys, successes, failures, regrets and the People who are most important to You".

COL

"I offer You one solemn promise. I will do my very best to insure that You will not perish from this world without another Human Heart beating at your side."

COL

BEN

▲ ▲ ▲

I WAS CONTACTED BY THE Volunteer Coordinator at Hospice of the Monterey Peninsula to see if I would be willing to take on a fairly unique assignment. Ben was an 88 year old man suffering with advanced small cell carcinoma lung cancer. He had been admitted to Hospice recently and was not expected to survive for very many weeks. He had lost his Wife of almost sixty years of marriage to cancer several years before. He was living with his Son Jamie in a private home residence in Monterey, California. Though Ben had two other Adult Children, they lived in other states and were not able to provide any practical means of day-to-day care.

I was told that this was expected to be a "Respite Visit". I met with Ben and Jamie during my initial visitation. Ben was bed-ridden in an electric hospital bed positioned in the central living room. He seemed to be very lethargic and barely cognizant of his surroundings. He generally appeared to sleep most of the time. However, he was calm and comfortable. Jamie explained to me that he had given Ben medication to help him remain relaxed and at ease.

Jamie explained to me that he had to work during the day to earn the income necessary to maintain the household. With Ben's health failing, the Family was at a loss as how to best deal with their difficult situation. Hospice Staff could help somewhat. The visiting Nurse would come by two to three times each week and the Home Health Aide would visit on almost a daily basis to provide hands-on care. Also, as a Volunteer I could become one small piece of the overall strategy to deliver the "best care possible" under the circumstances.

So, I was asked to come by once a week and visit and check in on Ben when no one else was actually in the house. I was to go to the side of the house, enter the back yard through a gate and then enter the house through a sliding glass door in the back. So, in subsequent visits, this was my routine. I would spend about two hours there at Ben's bedside. Sometimes he was awake and aware of my presence and at other times he was asleep. I always had Jamie's phone number on hand in case I needed to communicate with him. Each of my visits there were uneventful. Ben always appeared calm and out of pain. When possible I would gently talk with him about simple subjects. Sometimes I read quietly to him. Other times I remained silent.

My specialized visitations went on for about five weeks only. Then I was informed by the Agency that Ben had passed with his Son at his side. The Family had expressed tremendous appreciation for the Hospice Agency and Staff providing critical circumstantial support during this tumultuous time. It is noteworthy that Jamie and the rest of Ben's Family placed tremendous trust with Hospice and the various personnel engaged with Ben at the End-of-Life. As a Volunteer, I was assigned the extraordinary task of venturing into a stranger's house to provide compassion and companionship to a stranger engaged in a desperate struggle. These types of assignments are profoundly satisfying.

CHAPTER 11

FRIENDLY VISITOR

▲ ▲ ▲

OVERVIEW

As a Hospice Volunteer, the "Friendly Visitor" assignment generally entails traveling to the current living setting and situation of the Patient and spending time there as a friendly companion in conversation and various appropriate activities. The overall goal for such efforts is to promote the social and emotional well-being of the Patient. This is offered as an integral part of the total person approach to Hospice support. Friendly Volunteers can be sent into Private Homes, Assisted Living Facilities, smaller Board and Care dwellings, as well as into Skilled Nursing Facilities or even temporarily into Acute Care Hospitals.

Some Hospice Agencies offer other forms of specialized support through their "Friendly Visitor" programs. These may include such services as light housekeeping, cooking and serving meals, small repair and maintenance jobs, grocery shopping, picking up prescription medications, driving Patients to various appointments or taking them shopping, etc. Again, not every Hospice Agency across the country offers all these various services. As a new or experienced Volunteer, always check with your Coordinator as to which, if any of these support services your Agency offers within their own internal Policies and Procedures. Each of these expanded services necessitate some degree of training as well as tighter controls due to heightened liability issues.

The idea of the Hospice Agency providing such a friendly Volunteer is usually introduced to the Patient and Family during the initial interviews by the Admissions Nurse or the Social Worker. The question is put to Patients and Family Members whether or not they might enjoy the informal company of such trained Volunteers to visit, to reminisce or to engage in fun and stimulating activities. The Patient of course is under no obligation to receive such attention or support while receiving Hospice Care.

When the Patient does agree to have such a Visitor, that request is passed on to the Volunteer Coordinator who then offers the assignment to the pool of trained Volunteers through a variety of channels. The Coordinator will routinely update and email a list of current assignments to all Volunteers. Such Volunteers are then free to pick among these various current requests. Then they can ideally choose that assignment that best fits their personality, interests, temperament, time available and geography. In some instances, the Coordinator might contact an individual Volunteer to determine if that Volunteer might be willing to take on a specific assignment that seems to match well with a unique Patient.

As a Volunteer Friendly Visitor, You are considered by the Agency as a vital member of the Interdisciplinary Team or Group (IDT-IDG). With your on-going visits, You provide a unique service to the overall welfare and Quality-of-Life of both Patient and Family Members. It is recognized by the Team that in End-of-Life Care, there is enormous therapeutic value in social engagement. You also serve as an extra "set of eyes" on the conditions and attitudes and moods of Patient and Family as they change over time. You provide observations and information through your regular reports back to the Agency in the form of "Activity Logs". This input is included by your Volunteer Coordinator in the regular IDT-IDG assessments of each Patient conducted by your Agency. The reports and details of your interactions with Patient and Family become a permanent part of the Patient's medical records.

Also, your Volunteer activity is precisely recorded and analyzed to calculate the critical 5% Rule required by Medicare (and Medicaid) for Agencies receiving Hospice compensation. Your travel time and mileage may also factor into this calculation. This is why your Coordinator will strongly encourage You to file your Activity Log Reports accurately and in a timely fashion. Your Agency is required to maintain such records currently for regular state or federal inspections or surveys.

PRIOR TO THE FIRST VISIT

Once You and your Volunteer Coordinator have agreed on a Friendly Visitor assignment, it is valuable for You to collect certain information about the Patient, the surrounding Loved Ones and the situation You will be encountering. Oftentimes, You and the Coordinator might initially discuss the central aspects of the case over the phone. Thereafter the Agency will forward the "Case Sheet" or "Face Sheet" to You via email or regular mail detailing the assignment.

These basic information sheets usually include the following facts.

* Patient's ID Number or Case Number.
* Patient's name, age, gender, phone number, living "setting" as in Private Home, Assisted Living Facility, Skilled Nursing Facility, etc.
* Patient's marital status, race or ethnicity, religious affiliation if any, primary language.
* Primary Medical Diagnosis – This is generally the medical condition for which the Patient has been placed into a "Hospice Status"; this is the underlying disease which is expected to eventually cause the Patient's death.
* Secondary Medical Diagnoses – This will list other significant formal diagnoses that may have a significant impact on the Patient's daily physical or cognitive conditions.
* Patient's primary personal Caregiver or important Social Support Network and phone number contacts.
* Relevant Hospice Agency personnel assigned to the case; this incudes Attending Physician, Case Manager, visiting Nurse, Social Worker, Chaplain or Spiritual Counselor, Home Health Aide, etc.

As a Hospice Volunteer going into a new Assignment for the first time, there are several other critical issues You will want to address. Your Volunteer Coordinator should be able to provide this expanded information or to refer You to the Agency's assigned Case Manager or Social Worker to better prepare You for your initial visit. These issues include the following topics.

* <u>Patient's Functional Status:</u> Are Patients safely "ambulatory"? Can they walk unassisted or perhaps with the aid of a cane or walker? Can they go to the bathroom without help? Are they confined to a bed? Can they eat and drink without restrictions? Are they continent or do they routinely wear adult diapers? Can they follow spoken words and can they speak coherently? Can they be taken outside for a brief walk?

* <u>Patient's Cognitive Status:</u> To what degree are Patients "alert and oriented" to their surroundings? This generally encompasses the four factors of being cognizant of "Person, Place, Time and Circumstance". Do they understand clearly "who" they are talking with, "where" they are presently, what approximately is the current "time and day and date", and what their overall "situation" is? Does the Patient have any history of forgetfulness or mental confusion? Does the Patient have a diagnosis of "Mild Cognitive Impairment", or any "Dementia" or even "Alzheimer's Disease"? If so, how severe are the behavioral symptoms of these conditions? How will they impact a routine friendly visit?

* <u>Patient's other Medical Issues:</u> Does the Patient also have other significant conditions that may impact the course and duration of a friendly visit? Do Patients suffer with Arthritis, Diabetes, Respiratory Disease, Paralysis, Neurological Disorders, Hearing or Seeing Problems, etc.

* <u>Patient's Social Network:</u> Besides the Patient, exactly whom will the Hospice Volunteer encounter and deal with during the visitation? What is that Person's connection to the Patient? Will that

contact remain at the house during the visit or will that Person leave (Respite visit)? That Individual should be able to explain many practical and important details about the Patient's current circumstances.

* Patient's preferred time and day to visit: Does the Patient or surrounding Family have any specific preferences about the day of the week or time of the day for a visitation? Is the Patient more energetic and engaging in the morning or afternoon? Are there regularly scheduled appointments with Hospice Agency personnel, such as the Home Health Aide or Visiting Nurse that the friendly visit should be planned around?

* Patient's Abilities and Interests: Does the Patient have well known interests and abilities that various activities might be planned around? Or, will the present plan for visitation simply be sitting quietly with the Patient?

These additional pieces of information and insight concerning the circumstances around a Patient are vital to a meaningful initial friendly visit. The more knowledge the Volunteer has approaching each visit, the more effective that visit should be for all parties.

THE FRIENDLY VISIT

The length of Volunteer Hospice assignments can range from "zero" days to several months. Once in a while You will agree to take on a new assignment and later be informed by your Agency that the Patient has already passed away, before your initial visit. You see them zero times. Most assignments will last several weeks or even over several months. You need to understand and be willing at the outset to take on such a commitment. When going into a private "home setting", You will generally be visiting at a regularly scheduled time and day, at least once a week. Visits can run from around ½ hour to perhaps two hours, depending on the condition and energy of the Patient. As a Volunteer it is important for You to understand how profound and important these assignments are to the Patient and Family. You are becoming an integral part of their life stories during a tumultuous and often desperate time.

It will be helpful for You, the Friendly Visitor, to keep in mind that every Patient You see and every visit You go on is unique. You will never know exactly quite what You might encounter with each new visit. Your experience during your next meeting may be very similar to your last visit, or it may be fundamentally different. Although there is a "social element" to your visits, a Hospice friendly visit is really not merely a "social engagement". There are several critical factors that are very different from a casual, friendly meeting with acquaintances. Again, in Hospice Care, the Patient and surrounding Loved Ones are caught up in the overwhelming and confusing and depressing confrontation with a life-shortening disease. Their most basic priorities and time-line horizons about their lives have shifted dramatically. They are often being driven on an intense roller coaster of emotional ups and downs that can change in an instant. The anticipated course for the Patient is one of inevitable decline, incapacity and death. This is the profound and desperate underlying Human situation that You as a Friendly Visitor are "wading" into. Again, this is hardly a normal social outing.

And yet, paradoxically as a Hospice representative, You are there precisely to attempt to bring the positive emotional Human benefit of a friendly social interaction. Ideally, this can have a powerful therapeutic effect on the Patient's current well-being. The more assignments and experience You, as a Hospice Volunteer go through, the more confident You will become about each visitation.

After compiling all the relevant information from your Agency about the Patient's conditions, including the close Family Caregivers, and the situations You will be encountering, You will then contact the Family directly by phone. During this initial conversation, You should review briefly the key medical information You have received from the Agency. You will also ask about the best day of the week and time of the day to visit. Confirm exactly who will be there and who will remain there during the visit. Ask about what kinds of activities, if any the Patient might be interested in doing during the visit. Also, it is generally a good idea to tell the Family that You will call an hour or two before the actual visit to remind them that You will be there. Going forward, some Families will ask You to place such a call before every visit. Other Families will tell You that they will expect You at your scheduled time and that You do not need to call before each visit. Just do exactly as they request.

It is extremely important for You to be reliable in terms of the Patient's and Family's expectations of your visits. Again, keep in mind that they are under intense emotional pressure and stress because of the situation they are enduring. It is a relatively minor issue, but it is helpful if they can depend on your promises and efforts from one week to the next. If for any reason You will be substantially late or unable to make an expected visit, You need to always call them ahead of time. During this conversation You should confirm your later expected time of arrival if running late, or the time and day of your next scheduled visit. Also, for a variety of reasons, there may be cases where the Family may cancel a visit through the Agency and this information will be relayed to You. Likewise, the Family may cancel a visit for various reasons during your confirmation call before stopping by. You truly need to make it a "habit" of being regarded as highly dependable by the Patient and Family Members.

As a friendly visiting Hospice Volunteer, You should quickly develop a critical social "skill or ability" to utilize whenever You encounter a Patient and surrounding Loved Ones. You will learn to automatically "assume a neutral emotional and energetic attitude" towards the Patient, towards individual Loved Ones and to the overall situation You are encountering. This means that You will go into each new or next assignment without any planned emotional agenda or expectations of what will occur during the visitation. You need to be aware of and "match" the emotional and energetic environment You find yourself within. (Note-this is fundamentally different from tentatively planning various "activities" during an upcoming visit.)

So, for example, You will sometimes walk into a situation where there is funny, friendly laughter and storytelling going on. In this case, You discover that both Patient and Family Members are in an active and positive mood. It is important for You to "assume" a similar attitude and behavior. If You walk in with a sullen, sorrowful or depressed frame of mind, it will contradict the emotional energy in the room. Similarly, if You go in to visit a Patient and You deliberately try to take on a light-hearted and humorous mind-set, and the Patient and Loved Ones are feeling overwhelmed and angry and confused, You may well come across as insensitive or dismissive of their circumstances.

Again, You should approach each new and next visitation with a conscious "neutral emotional and energetic attitude" and then adjust your personal perspectives and behavior to reflect the circumstances You encounter. This is an innate Human empathic ability You will develop and perfect with each new assignment.

You should endeavor to be as prepared as is possible for each new or next visit. Always try to have in mind what you "might" engage in before each visitation. (Again, this is different from the planned "neutral emotional engagement" talked about above.) Using the general information from your Agency and in speaking with Family Members, during your first visit, You will probably simply plan on friendly introductions and getting to know each other. This obviously assumes that the Patient is still capable of coherent conversation and social interactions. During subsequent visits, You might dig deeper into biographical questions and reminiscing about the Patient's life, relationships and interests. Depending on the Patient's present mood and energy, You might pick from the *"Activities Sheet"* and be prepared to engage in something that might be of interest. Approaching and even during a Hospice visit, You will always need to be highly flexible and ready and willing to change plans and Activities based upon the Patient's conditions. You might go in planning to engage in a specific activity, but upon arrival realize that the Patient does not have the energy nor inclination to do so. You will simply adjust your efforts accordingly. Also, it is often the case that the most meaningful role You can play is to be a quiet compassionate presence with little or no verbal communication.

As mentioned, the actual course and duration of each friendly visit will depend primarily upon the Patient's current physical and mental conditions. During one week's encounter, the Patient may be energetic, active and in a good mood. The following week, You may find the Patient tired, distracted, sleepy and depressed. Again, You will learn to quickly adjust to whatever You run into. The more times You visit the Patient and Family, the better will be your understanding and insights about the overall situation.

As a Hospice Volunteer, it will be helpful for You to be mindful of the Human realities You are dealing with. You are involved with a Patient who is on an inexorable dying trajectory. Whether You spend several weeks or several months visiting that Individual, during that time-frame, You will remain generally stable and healthy. However, You will be involved as a first-hand witness to that Person's gradual incapacity and death. This will require an inevitable readjustment to continual change on your part. This is the common pattern in End-of-Life care.

CHAPTER 12

INTERACTIONS WITH FAMILY AND LOVED ONES

▲ ▲ ▲

WHEN YOU PERFORM WORK AS a Friendly Visitor, You will often interact with the Patient's surrounding "social network" at some point. This network is referred to generically as "Family Members and Loved Ones". This can include a wide range of Individuals who have some connection with the Patient. It <u>encompasses each Person that the Patient regards as a close, meaningful Human companion in life.</u> It might include a Spouse, Ex-Spouse, Partner, Adult and Young Children, Step-Children, Grandchildren, Greatgrandchildren, Siblings, Aunts, Uncles, Cousins and of course Close Friends. Over the course of a lifetime, the Patient may well have many such relationships.

As the Hospice Patient draws closer to the End-of-Life, these various relationships usually take on profound new perspectives and meanings. The process of declining and dying affects not only the Patients' experiences, but also that of those Individuals that care about them. Exactly how these caring Individuals react to the prospect of impending death can vary a great deal. Reactions can be affected by circumstances. A Spouse living with a dying Spouse will be impacted completely. A Cousin who was close to the dying Patient during childhood, but who has resided in another state for many years will be affected differently. A small child of a Patient will generally react differently from an older Adult Child. A close Friend will respond differently from a church Associate.

The reactions of Individuals within the Patient's social network can also vary widely based on the emotional connections and closeness of the relationships with the Patient. Usually the stronger and more engaged the connection to the Patient is, the stronger will be the impact of immanent death on surrounding Family Members and Loved Ones.

However, different People will respond differently to the specter of a death. Human Beings deal with the subject and the reality of death in very different ways. Some People can barely bring themselves to think about it, let alone being in the presence or being involved with a dying Person. Most People have no idea about how to behave around or what to say to a terminally ill Individual. Some fear that they may do or say something inappropriate, insensitive, confrontational or out of place. So, when the news about a Hospice Patient gets around to the immediate and more distant social network, there will typically be a wide range of responses. Some People will seem to step forward and try to offer practical help, while Others will seem to fade away. Even those that would usually be regarded as closest to the Patient may act in very differing manners. Some Siblings or Adult Children will offer active support and seek to intervene on a regular basis, while Others may barely remain in contact with the Patient. Some Family Members or Loved Ones may feel compelled to "orchestrate" or "control" the decisions and course of on-going care. Still Others may be at a complete loss as to how to proceed and offer no ideas or opinions. Some may be rendered numb, while Others cannot stop directing things.

Due to the intensity and complexity of these situations, it is often the case that many disagreements and conflicts can arise among the various Family Members and Loved Ones. Some may remain entrenched in "denial" of the original life-threatening disease diagnosis. They may press for a second or third medical opinion. They may try to insist that any possible treatment protocol must be pursued. They feel that a "never give up" attitude must be maintained. Still, Others may quickly acquiesce to the perceived inevitability of the diagnosis and try to plan for life accordingly.

Perhaps the most difficult challenges arise when there is a distinct difference between the Patient's changing perspectives and those of various Members of the social network. Within the "five stage frame work" of Kubler-Ross, the Patient may have progressed into an "acceptance" attitude, while well-meaning Loved Ones may still be in "denial" and pressing for further clinical testing or medical treatments. The Patient may privately feel exhausted and overwhelmed by the long struggle and may simply want to be made comfortable, left alone and let nature take its course. Family Members may not be emotionally ready to embrace such passivity and may want the fight to continue. If Family Members have never really experienced the death of a close Loved One, they may not be capable of accepting the inevitability of this death.

Again, as a Friendly Visitor, You will normally encounter various Members of the Patient's social network during your regular visits. This is especially true when your visitations occur within a "private home setting". You may not meet the entire surrounding network. In fact, there may be many Members that are very close to the Patient that You never interact with at all. Keep in mind, that in general You spend only two to three hours per week in the presence of the Patient. You only witness a brief "snapshot" of the Patient's life, including mood, energy, cognitive status and environment at that specific time. For the most part, You will be unaware of everything that has transpired since your previous visit. You will only have access to knowledge about the changing situation through your brief observations and the information that the Patient and Family choose to reveal to You. If You are visiting a Patient within an Assisted Living Facility or Skilled Nursing Facility, You will usually have no input from Loved Ones.

However, it is extremely important for You to keep in mind what your overall objectives are during each visit. <u>You are there in the vital role of a kind, empathic, compassionate Friendly Visitor. You are there to engage the Patient in whatever kinds of conversation or activities that Patient finds enjoyable or meaningful at the time.</u> You are not there as a Therapist. You are not there as a Spiritual Counselor. You are not there as a Medical Professional. You are not there to solve their problems. Likewise, You are not there to resolve any conflicts they may have with individual Members of their social network. You can and should listen to any comments or complaints the Patient may offer concerning other People. (If You regard these conflicts as significant, You should communicate these issues confidentially to your Agency Coordinator, Case Manager or Social Worker.) However, You should never take it upon yourself to attempt to remedy these issues.

The difficult and often tumultuous events surrounding the dying and death of an Individual within Hospice Care usually involve multiple People. Death is most often a community event. Various Family Members and Loved Ones are inextricably caught up by circumstances and emotional connections to the Patient. Individuals react to this profound situation in many different ways. Some step up and become closely involved, while Others fade away. As a Friendly Visitor, You will often witness many of these issues first hand. You simply need to stay mindful of the specific roles You are there to fulfill and do your best to do so.

CHAPTER 13

VOLUNTEER INTERACTION WITH PATIENTS AND FAMILY WITHIN VARIOUS "HOME SETTINGS"

▲ ▲ ▲

AS DESCRIBED BEFORE, FORMAL HOSPICE support is offered into a multitude of Patient "home settings". These include Private Residences, Assisted Living Facilities, Skilled Nursing Facilities and even on occasion, Acute Care Hospitals. As a Hospice Volunteer, your interaction with Patients and surrounding Loved Ones will vary a great deal due to the "home setting" location You are visiting. Each "setting" requires a different approach and strategy.

When You go to a <u>Private Residence</u>, You are entering a personal private living space. This is their home base and has generally been that way for a long time. You have been invited in as a "guest". It is important that You treat the Patient and all close Loved Ones You encounter with the utmost respect. You must keep in mind that they are all enduring a calamitous and desperate situation. Within their midst, they are coping with a gradual and inexorable loss of one of their most precious Human treasures. You will find that their moods and behaviors may change drastically from one day or week to the next. During one visit, You may witness the Patient and Family Members being jovial and laughing and telling stories. During the follow-up visit, the overall mood be one of anger and sadness and confusion. You may find that the Patient is calm and dreamy, while a Loved One may feel overcome with fatigue and depression.

As You gain more and more experience, You will learn to be even-tempered and supportive in whatever kind of emotional environments

You may walk into. (Recall the "neutral emotional-energy" attitude You should assume when going into your first or your next visitation). Remember, You are not there to resolve their problems. You are not there to correct their attitudes. You are not there to get Loved Ones to feel better or become happy or accepting of the situation. You have no capacity to alter the Patient's medical conditions. You are there simply as a Hospice Volunteer in the role of a Friendly Visitor. They may want to simply "vent" their fear and anguish. They may want to express anger or shed tears. They may want to tell You touching stories about their Loved Ones. The Patient may want to review the latest sports scores, or relate their old war stories. They may want to watch their favorite TV shows. They may want to listen to music or have You read to them. They may want to remain completely silent. The activities that are meaningful at that moment will be determined by the Patient and Family. They will not be directed by You. You are simply the friendly Patient companion there to offer your time and attention and to act as a compassionate listener and conversationalist. But, sooner or later, You will realize that there is enormous value in what You are doing.

In general, when You are visiting a Patient and Family in a Private Resident, You will need to set up a routine day and time to visit that accommodates their situation. You should make all efforts to maintain that schedule. During your initial visit to their home, You should ask if they would prefer You to call each week to remind them of your impending visit. Some will say yes to this suggestion, while others will tell You that it is not necessary. If for some reason You cannot make a regular scheduled visit, You should call and inform the Family of the change. The Patient and surrounding Loved Ones are going through an intense and often chaotic time and You need to be sensitive and respectful to their circumstances.

When You are going into an <u>Assisted Living Facility</u>, the approach and routine may be very different from when You visit Patients and Family in their own private homes. In general, ALFs are large and complex facilities with many Residents and a large staff of workers to sustain the operation. Individual Residents living there are usually in their own private living quarters. This can be a simple room with a bed, furniture, TV, perhaps a refrigerator and stove. It might also be a fully furnished individual apartment dwelling with multiple rooms. Residents may live within these units alone or with a Spouse or Partner. ALFs usually have a large central dining area where Residents can go for all meals. Residents can also have meals delivered to their rooms. The facilities offer a wide range of support services which Residents can pick and choose from for their daily routines. Residents are also provided with assistance with "activities of daily living" (ADLs) as needed. ALFs also provide a large variety of activities which Residents can participate in if desired. These can include musical performances, arts and crafts, religious services, movies, etc.

When You visit one of these large facilities, You may be asked to "sign in" and then "sign out" at a central lobby or desk area. Some facilities will be very strict about this, while others are not so. Just do whatever they ask You to do. Remember, You are there as a professional representative of your Agency. Make sure You act accordingly. As always, make sure You are wearing your ID badge identifying You and the Hospice Agency You work for.

Unless You are visiting a Patient living with a Spouse or Partner, You will usually be seeing that Person in a one-on-one basis. This means that You will usually not be encountering Family or Loved Ones. When You approach the door of the room of the Patient You are there to visit, always knock and announce Yourself. Do not simply walk in. For example, You knock and say loudly, "This is Craig, I am with Vitas, and I am here to see John". Wait a minute or more and repeat the process. Repeat it a third time. It is often the case that the Patient may be hard of hearing, may not be very mobile or may even be asleep. If there is still no answer, open the door slightly and announce again who you are and why you are there. Only then should You step into the room and try to determine what is going on. Announce again who You are, but at some distance away from the Resident. Try to not startle or scare the Resident by suddenly being next to the person. If the Resident is sound asleep, You might quietly call the Person's name a couple of times and see if that wakes the Individual up. If it does not, You might consider letting them sleep and plan on coming back at another time. This will be a judgement call on your part.

Sometimes during a visitation, a Facility Staff Member may come in to administer medications or bring in a snack. You generally do not need to leave the room. If staff are there to perform some kind of hands-on care, You might step out for a few minutes. Try to avoid visiting at mealtimes. After a couple of visits try to determine what time of day is best for You to visit.

It is sometimes the case that exactly "when" You visit may be somewhat more flexible with a Patient living in an ALF, than going into a private home with Family Members also living there. When going into a private setting, surrounding Loved Ones usually plan on your arrival at a specific day and time of the week. When visiting a Patient one-on-one in a facility, it is more reasonable to be able to visit in the "mornings" or "afternoons" sometime during the week. Obviously, if the Patient does ask for a specific day and time, You do your best to comply with that request. Otherwise, You do have some practical flexibility about when You visit.

The exception to the larger facility described above is the so-called "Board and Care" facility which houses six or less Residents. Generally, these are large single family homes that have been converted into and licensed as an Assisted Living Facility. When You go to one of these locations, You may or may not actually meet the "owner" of the facility. You may deal only with the small staff working there. These facilities generally have the feel of a large family community. Residents may have a private room or they may share a room with a roommate. You will generally be visiting with the Patient on a one-on-one basis. Similar to larger ALFs, You will usually not be interacting directly with Family or Loved Ones. You might ask the staff to help You find a quiet corner within the facility in which You can talk with the Patient.

Similar to larger ALF visitations, You should have more flexible leeway in terms of when You visit a Patient living in the typical Board and Care. You might visit during mornings or afternoons, depending on at what time of the day the Patient is more energetic or receptive to visitors. As always, plan your activity during the visit. Assume the "neutral emotional and energy" going in. Be observant and let the Patient's conditions determine the length and course of the visit.

The experience of visiting a Patient living in a <u>Skilled Nursing Facility</u> will usually be very different from those described above. In general, You will be walking into a very busy and complex medicalized setting. This will usually include a central lobby area, multiple wings of rooms, Nurses' stations, central dining and activity areas, busy Nurses, Nurses' Assistants, Dieticians, Social Workers, Activity Directors, kitchen and laundry Workers, Janitors and various Administrative Personnel. Again, whether Patients are there in temporary rehab or living in permanent custodial care, they are there because a Physician has certified that they require 24-hour nursing care.

Some facilities may be strict about having You sign in and out in the front lobby, while others will not. Always do whatever they ask You to do. It is especially important for You to always wear your ID badge so that others will know exactly who You are and why You are present within this busy and complex operation. Sometimes the Patient You visit will be in a single room with no roommate. However, it is usually the case that your Patient will be sharing a room with one or even two Residents. You will generally be visiting without any Family Members or Loved Ones present. Remember the "neutral emotional-energy" attitude when approaching each Patient. If your Patient's room door is closed, knock and announce who You are and who You are with. Do this at least three times before You quietly open the door, step inside and repeat your announcement. Take quick stock of your Patient and of any other Residents in the room. Always be quiet and respectful if anyone appears to be asleep. Approach your Patient gently. If they seem to be asleep, call their name three times to see if they wake up. If they remain asleep, it might be better to try to visit at another time.

Your Patient will very often be confined to the bed. Always try to get a chair so that You will sit with your eyes at their eye level. The kinds of activities You bring to the Patient will be similar to those of any Hospice visit. You may ask biographical questions, ask about their school, work, Loved Ones, military service, hobbies, interests, etc. You may bring their favorite music to play. You may read to them. You may go through a photo album, etc. Always be aware of the Patient's mood and energy level. Be very careful to not exhaust them. If they appear to grow weary, politely end the visit. Again, You are there as a friendly, patient, compassionate companion.

As a Hospice Volunteer, You may actually be called upon to visit Patients suffering with progressive and advanced forms of <u>Dementia or Alzheimer's Disease</u> in all settings. In other words, You may encounter such Patients in a <u>Private Residence, Assisted Living Facility,</u> including a <u>Board and Care,</u> and in a <u>Skilled Nursing Facility.</u> (Refer to the chapter on Cognitive decline within Hospice Care) In some larger ALFs and SNFs, there may be a separate and secure wing or ward where Dementia sufferers are cared for. Exactly how You engage these Patients will be a reflection of the settings they live in.

There can be a wide variety of the severity and associated behaviors of these afflictions. Your on-going visits and interactions with these Patients will be unique and individually tailored to each. With some, You might utilize common activities such as asking questions about their life, work, family, etc. For others, playing music may prove more appropriate. Still for others, the most effective connection may simply be holding hands and saying nothing. As a Hospice Volunteer, your underlying goal is always to try to determine what is most meaningful to the Patient You are visiting.

You will gradually and inevitably become more comfortable and gain more confidence with each new assignment and every individual visit. This encompasses each of the "home settings" described above.

CHAPTER 14

RESPITE VISITS

▲ ▲ ▲

"RESPITE" SUPPORT IS A VERY important and specialized form of a Hospice Friendly visit. In this case, the Volunteer stays with the Patient while Family or Loved Ones who routinely live with and care for that Patient temporarily leave. The Family Member or Loved One withdraws from the immediate situation of being physically and emotionally engaged with the Patient. The Hospice goal is to provide Loved Ones short-term "respite from" the work and pressures of caregiving. For many Family Members, this serves as a vital form of caring support offered at a critical phase of their trying situation.

Family Members will usually leave the premises to pursue a variety of common activities. They may run errands, go to the bank or the gym or the park. They may go shopping or to various scheduled appointments. They may attend church services. They may walk the dog or visit friends. They may simply retire into a secluded room within the house, or move to another location on the property. Again, the key is to give Caregivers a brief mental and emotional break from the stress of the difficult circumstances they are coping with on a daily basis.

Respite visits may be a one-time request. Family or Loved Ones may have a special event to attend and they want the Patient cared for by someone they trust. On the other hand, Respite visitations may be carried on at a regularly scheduled time and day of the week for an extended period of time. Individual visitations will generally last one or two and sometimes three hours. Respite support is usually only meaningful within a "private home setting", where close Family Members live with and care for the Patient. In an Assisted Living Facility or Skilled Nursing Facility, regular Staff Members will be on hand to provide care.

Identical to any other Hospice Friendly Visit, You should endeavor to obtain as much information as possible about the Patient and the situation You will be encountering. This includes functional and cognitive and medical status. It also encompasses developing a tentative approach to any meaningful activities You might engage in during your visit. In practical terms, You will naturally acquire very critical information and insights from the Family Members You will meet during your first visit. You should have a reasonably clear understanding of what to expect, what is permissible and safe as well as what is not permissible and not safe during your time there.

So for example, You might ask whether or not You are allowed to give the Patient any foods or liquids during the visit. What is expected of You if the Patient needs to get out of bed and go the bathroom? Are You allowed to take the Patient out for a walk or to sit outside on a porch? What if the Patient asks for pain medication while You are there? If any urgent situation occurs, You can seek out guidance from either the Family Member or Your Agency via phone contact.

During Respite Visits, it is absolutely necessary for You to initially gather key "contact information" about the Family Members for whom You are providing respite. In other words, if a routine or an emergency question were to come up during your visit, exactly how will You get hold of that Family Member in real time? During your introductory meeting with the Patient and Family Caregiver, You must collect that Family Member's cell phone and confirm that You have it stored correctly. This must be available for any event in which You need to ask the Caregiver an immediate question. In the case that the Family Member does not carry a cell phone, some other Family contact number must be obtained.

As always, it is the case that You will keep on hand all relevant phone numbers of key Staff Members of your Hospice Agency. Also, your Agency will of course have Physician and Nursing support by phone 24/7.

So, even on nights or weekends, You will always have close phone live support if You need it. Again, as a Hospice Volunteer working in the field, You are never really alone.

Your basic approach to any Respite Visit should be similar to any other Friendly Visit. Collect as much information as possible. Plan possible Activities. Assume a "neutral emotional and energetic" perspective going in. Be flexible and patient. During your time there, You will be providing an extraordinary service to both Patient and Loved Ones in very extraordinary times.

CHAPTER 15

VIGIL VOLUNTEER

▲ ▲ ▲

A "VIGIL" IS A SERVICE offered by most Hospice Agencies to Patients and Loved Ones. It entails providing a constant Human caring "presence" to be with an actively dying Person at the very End-of-Life. This on-going attention and support is generally provided by a team of trained Volunteers taking turns being at the bedside of the Patient during this most difficult and yet profound experience.

Even though, as mentioned before, it is virtually impossible to predict the exact day and time at which a Patient will die, there are several conditions and behaviors that indicate death is very near. Patients may become extremely weak and sleep (be unconscious) most of the time. They may have recently refused any food or fluids intake. They may have displayed some degree of cognitive "confusion". They may show discoloration or coldness in their extremities. Their pulse rate may have become irregular. Their breathing may have become shallow, irregular and even intermittent. These are all common indicators that the end may be at hand.

Concerned Family Members and Loved Ones may request Vigil support for a variety of reasons. The most common reason is that Loved Ones simply do not want the dying Person to be alone during this dramatic stage of life. Sometimes the individual Family Members live some distant away, have pressing obligations they must take care of before coming to the Patient's bedside, or are unable to visit the dying Person due to the Loved One's medical or functional or cognitive problems.

Given the basic support goals of a Vigil assignment, It may seem curious to You as a Volunteer that sometimes Family or Loved Ones may remain present during your visit. This can be due to a variety of reasons. Family Members may simply feel better if a Hospice Person is present during this trying time. They may also want a personal option to be able to leave or disengage from the situation for a brief period of time and yet not leave their dying Loved One alone. If Family Members are there, You might gently see if they want to engage in conversation with You. If not, then silence is perfectly fine. As a Volunteer, You are there to try your very best to adapt and be a compassionate and caring presence no matter what the circumstances. You bring your common Human Self and heart and reverence and respect into this rarified arena.

Again, when supported within Hospice, the Patient is usually calm and quiet and asleep at the point of passing. For surrounding Family Members, the final transition in the Human life of a Loved One is often the most difficult, painful, surreal, desperate, sorrowful experience possible. For others, it may be "spiritual" or profound or the natural ending within the circle of life.   The reaction of Family Members may be very different if the dying Person is a child as compared to the passing of a 90 year old Individual.

Vigil support can be readily provided wherever the Patient's current "home setting" is. This can be a Private Residence, Senior Living Community, Assisted Living Facility, free standing, In-Patient Hospice location, Skilled Nursing Facility or even an Acute Care Hospital. Wherever Patients are spending their last moments, a Vigil Volunteer will be there if requested.

<u>As it is difficult or impossible to predict the exact time of death, it is also difficult to anticipate when a Patient may quickly transition into the process of actively dying.</u> Therefore, Hospice Agencies must be organized to react to the changing conditions of Patients very quickly. Vigil Volunteers must be trained and on call, ready to consider or accept a Vigil assignment when it suddenly presents itself. Due to the pressing nature of the situation, Agencies will generally send out a text or email to

Volunteers with the description and "time-frames" needed or available to provide Vigil support to a specific Patient. Some Agencies offer 24-hour support, while others offer 8:00am to 10:00pm support. Assignments are usually given in two hour "segments". So, a Volunteer might take the assignment to be at the Patient's bedside between 2:00pm to 4:00pm each day until the Person passes away. Obviously, the Volunteer is free to pick and choose whatever time slots are available at the time. The overall process of filling all the assignments will be coordinated through the Agency Volunteer Coordinator or Assistant. The Vigil services will generally continue until the Patient passes away.

Agencies that offer Vigil Services will usually require prospective Volunteers to go through a specialized Training Program. Such a program may include two to four hours of extra education focused on providing caring support for Patients and Family at the very End-of-Life. Such support can be very different from the various forms of activities in which Volunteers usually engage.

Being a Vigil Volunteer can be some of the most challenging and heartfelt and yet fulfilling work You will ever do. It puts You within the stark Human realities of the death of a Person and the grieving Family as they witness the vanishing away of their Loved One. In the Human scheme of things, there is nothing more difficult or profound.

CHAPTER 16

PATIENTS WITH COGNITIVE DEFICITS

▲ ▲ ▲

ALTHOUGH THERE WILL ALWAYS BE exceptions, as a Hospice Friendly Visitor, You will usually be spending time with elderly Individuals. This is due to the fact that, the vast majority of Americans who are certified for Hospice Care are 65 years of age and older. The older a Person gets, the more susceptible that Individual is to serious illnesses. In medical terminology, "increasing age" is a primary "risk factor" for serious and eventually terminal diseases.

Also, as a Volunteer, You will be involved with many older Individuals who are suffering with a variety of "cognitive deficits". Likewise, "increasing age" is a primary "risk factor" for such cognitive decline. As Americans continue to enjoy a longer Life Expectancy, more and more end up with cognitive problems. Similar to other acute medical conditions, these Seniors simply live long enough to develop cognitive limitations. This means that, as a Friendly Visitor, You will be interacting directly with certain Individuals who are to some degree, mentally and emotionally confused and disoriented. These issues can create very difficult and unique challenges in any End-of-Life situations.

It is especially important for You as a Volunteer to develop a basic knowledge of the various patterns of Human cognitive decline. (See also the discussion on "cognitive issues" in the chapter on the Human Life Course.) It is helpful to describe such issues in terminology used by medical and psychological experts in their respective fields. The fundamental dimensions of Human cognitive experience can be best understood within the following parameters.

Memory: This encompasses an Individual's mental ability to acquire, store, retain and then be able to retrieve information about past experiences and events. The on-going continuity of a Person's memories form a basic component of that Individual's understanding and meaning and identity over the course of a lifetime. When assessing the complexities of Human cognitive decline, experts often use a "time-line" framework. Patients will be asked to recall details about certain personal memories within the following list.

* Immediate Memory: This describes the ability to retain immediate experiences. For example, if someone says three words to a Patient, that Patient can immediately repeat those three words back. A Person suffering severe cognitive problems may not be able to do so.

* Short-Term Memory: This entails the capacity to recall events that have occurred within the past few hours or days. For example, a Patient can easily remember the dinner menu from the previous night. Again, an Individual with cognitive problems may not be able to recall this simple fact.

* Intermediate Memory: This deals with the ability to readily remember experiences that occurred over the course of recent months or years. For example, a Patient is capable of recalling and describing work and career patterns over the last decade. Such recall may be difficult for a Person with impaired cognitive abilities.

* Long-term Memory: This encompasses the capacity to recall a life-time of accumulated memories going back to early childhood. For example, A Patient is able to describe the name of the teacher and the school from the fourth grade. A Person with serious cognitive loss may not be able to do so.

Orientation: This describes a Patient's present understanding of and engagement with the surrounding world. It is a very powerful and complex assessment of a Person's current cognitive status. It is usually organized into four components.

- Orientation to "Person": This refers to an Individual's recognition of the People within the immediate environment. In other words, a Patient recognizes Family Members or recalls the names of Caregivers. A Person suffering advanced cognitive problems may not recognize Loved Ones.
- Orientation to "Place": This deals with a Patient having a clear understanding of "where" that Person is at the present time. This means that a Person understands being at home or in a facility or a hospital. Again, when struggling with cognitive deficits, a Patient may lose track of the immediate environment.
- Orientation to "Time": This describes the understanding and awareness of the present "time-frame" the Patient is within. The Person will be able to tell what year or season or even day of the week that it is. A Patient enduring cognitive problems may not be able to talk about what time or day it currently is.
- Orientation to "Situation": This deals with being able to describe the overall circumstances and meaning of a Patient's current experiences. A Patient will have the capacity to detail why they are where they are and what is being done. A Patient with severe cognitive deficits may have no idea of what is going on around them or why certain things are happening.

So, for example, during a cognitive assessment, Patients may be described as being "Alert and Oriented X 4". This means that they are fully engaged and they comprehend the "real-world" circumstances of their environment. They do not appear to suffer from confusion nor hallucinations. They recognize the People around them, they know where they are, they understand their present time-frame, and they are cognizant of their overall reality.

Executive Function: This refers to a patient's intellectual ability to understand and analyze new information. It also includes the capacity to formulate specific plans and goals using this information. It encompasses connecting with learning experiences from the past in order to plan current and future actions. It is the ability to use abstract reasoning, evaluating and judging to develop strategic objectives and to then carry out plans to achieve them.

Cognitive Executive Function is utilized for very simple projects, as well as for extremely complex ones. For example, a Person may devise plans to rake the leaves and then cut the grass. Another Individual may spend several months developing a working automobile prototype. Both are relying on the same intellectual processes and skills.

So, Patients who suffer certain cognitive deficits may have difficulty with the exercise of Executive Function. They may struggle to draw on past learning, to integrate that learning with new information and to then be able to develop a future plan of action. Carrying out such a complicated intellectual activity may simply prove too difficult.

Understanding and Knowledge: This refers to the innate Human mental capacity for acquiring insight and learning about the world. It includes gaining meaningful knowledge and comprehension of various experiences. Psychologists refer to "crystallized intelligence" as the accumulation of various skills and understanding gathered over a lifetime. Likewise, they also refer to "fluid intelligence" as the continual acquisition of novel understanding and abilities. Together they describe the inherent Human capacity to learn about and to function meaningfully in the world.

Language and Communication: This deals with the processes of both verbal and written communications through language. Learning, retaining and using the abstract ideas and meanings within a language is enormously complex. It takes Humans a great deal of time and effort to become proficient in communicating through language. Again, Psychologists describe the ability to use language in two ways. "Receptive skills" refer to the capacity to comprehend both spoken and written words and ideas. "Expressive skills" deal with the ability to speak and write such words and ideas. Cognitive competence generally encompasses both skills.

Personality and Behaviors: This encompasses a wide range of multidimensional aspects of Human nature. Over a lifetime, Individuals develop and exhibit a variety of unique traits, characteristics, interests, abilities and valuations that make up One's personality. These factors are the results of complex interactions of genetic make-up and environmental influences. Generally, a Person's on-going behavioral engagements with the world is a reflection of this complicated process of personality. Individuals may be energetic, outgoing, intellectual, athletic, religious, timid, aggressive, nurturing, creative, compassionate, etc. Likewise, cognitive aspects of personality and affective behaviors may be judged to be healthy and balanced or they may be "problematic" or "pathological".

Using the above psychological parameters, Healthcare Professionals have developed a set of diagnostic concepts to define and delineate cognitive aging and decline in Humans. These include the following:

Normal Cognitive Aging: As Individuals mature into middle age and beyond, they naturally undergo a slowing down of some intellectual function and ability. An 85 year old Person does not learn or process information as effectively as a 20 year old does. However, this natural decline is generally regarded as a normal part of aging, if that Individual does not suffer dramatic deficits in "memory" or "orientation". Normal cognitive aging does not constitute a disease.

Mild Cognitive Impairment (MCI): This is the first medically recognized and diagnosed form of cognitive disease. It is most often associated with the onset of "short and intermediate term memory" problems. As such, it is more specifically defined as "amnestic mild cognitive impairment". A formal diagnosis requires extensive clinical tests and evaluations. In MCI, memory difficulties are assessed to be more severe than those that might occur with normal cognitive aging. However, a diagnosis of MCI does not include interference with routine "activities of daily living" (ADLs). In general, an Individual suffering with MCI is still able to carry on normal work and social routines.

Dementia: This is an umbrella term used by medical and psychological professionals to describe a wide range of cognitive deficits. It is the label that encompasses a complex group of "signs and symptoms" associated with a deterioration of cognitive ability and function. It is not a single condition or disease.

There are as many as 75 potential root "causes" of various dementias. In terms of medical assessment, diagnosis, treatment and prognosis, dementias are often classified as "reversible" or "irreversible". Examples can include conditions as diverse as Alzheimer's Disease, B-Vitamin deficiencies, brain tumors, kidney or liver disease, various infections, head injuries, drug allergies, Parkinson's Disease HIV or strokes.

"Reversible dementias" that manifest as mental confusion are generally temporary conditions that can be reversed or cured when the underlying cause or causes are addressed. These causes can include for example, a urinary tract infection (UTI), severe electrolyte imbalances, thyroid imbalances, liver infections, etc. Sometimes these short-term and curable dementias are described as "delirium".

"Irreversible dementias" are categorized as degenerative or progressive conditions. These include severe dementias that are medically irreversible, untreatable, incurable and ultimately fatal. These include such serious diseases as Alzheimer's Disease, ischemic vascular disease (from strokes), Lewy bodies dementia, frontotemporal dementia, corticobasal dementia, Huntington's disease, pugilistic dementia (so-called "boxer's syndrome" describing repeated trauma to the brain), as well as others.

These irreversible dementias are all "associated" with specific physiological conditions. They all include deterioration of various centers and structures within the brain. This means that certain portions of the brain will gradually atrophy over time. As brain cells or individual neurons die, neural pathways and connections are disrupted. In certain diseases such as Alzheimer's and Lewy Bodies dementia, this progressive process is associated with an abnormal accumulation of the so-called "amyloid plaques" and "neurofibrillary tangles" within the brain which leads to cell death. Researchers also associate certain forms of brain deterioration with insufficient blood circulation, severe inflammation, and even the buildup of so-called "free radicals" that cause damage to individual brain cells.

Dementias usually begin with minor difficulties with memory or recall of recent events and then progress to impact other cognitive dimensions. Again, it is often difficult to distinguish initially between the early stages of dementia and "normal cognitive aging". But, the more severe types of dementia are progressive in nature which means that they inevitably worsen as time goes on.

All of these forms of dementia manifest to various degrees as abnormal problems with one or more of the cognitive issues of "memory, orientation, executive function, understanding and communication". They can also manifest over time with fundamental changes in an Individual's "personality and behaviors". These cognitive difficulties and changes can range from very mild symptoms to total incapacitation. Again, not every sufferer experiences difficulties with each and every one of these cognitive factors.

Alzheimer's Disease is by far the most common form of severe dementia in the United States. There are approximately two and a half million Americans with a formal diagnosis of Alzheimer's Disease. Statistically, life expectancy following a formal medical diagnosis of Alzheimer's is over seven years. It is estimated that the total number of Individuals in this country suffering with various stages of Alzheimer's is around five million.

This means that virtually one in eight People in the United States over the age of 65 is enduring the gradual ravages of this disease.

The following "Case Studies" illustrate examples of Hospice Patients suffering various degrees of progressive dementias. Such cognitive deficits are usually in addition to other life-threatening conditions that warrant a formal Hospice or Palliative Care status. In some cases however, advanced stages of Alzheimer's Disease or other incurable dementias will be listed as the Primary Diagnosis leading to Hospice or Palliative Care status.

Edna: This is an 81 year old woman who taught high school math, was widowed 12 years ago, has three Adult Children, six Grandchildren and one Great-Grandchild. She was originally treated for breast cancer in her 40s, and was declared disease free. Now her cancer has returned and metastasized into her lungs, liver and lymph nodes. She has been on Hospice support for several weeks. She currently lives with her oldest Daughter and has a Home Health Aide come in five days a week while her Daughter works outside the house and Edna is alone. Over the past year, she has gradually become aware of increasing problems with her memory and her orientation to her environment. She has trouble recalling close Family Member's names. She forgets where she put things. She sometimes does not remember what she ate the previous night. Most alarming to her was when she found herself driving and could not recall where she was going. She has not yet been medically assessed for cognitive problems. However, she does appear to have the symptoms of early dementia.

Charles: This is a 66 year old man who worked construction for decades until he was severely injured on the job and went on permanent disability. He has suffered with respiratory ailments for several years. He was divorced at age 55 and had no children. He received a formal diagnosis of Chronic Obstructive Pulmonary Disease (COPD) at age 57. When he moved into his early 60s, his brother began to suspect that "Charles might have Alzheimer's, because he seems to be confused about simple stuff". His brother finally convinced him to undergo a psychological assessment and he was diagnosed with early onset "dementia" with unspecified causes. A close friend helped to get him into permanent residency within the "memory care" ward of an Assisted Living Facility. He has been living there for two years and his cognitive condition continues to worsen. He has withdrawn from most social engagements. He speaks very little and mumbles his words. He walks slowly with a distinct shuffle. He has to be helped with eating and toileting. His COPD has worsened to the point that he has been placed on Hospice Care.

Lorena: This is a 94 year old woman who was a wife and housekeeper for all of her adult life. She and her husband had seven children. Five made it to adulthood. She was widowed when she was 73. She remained active and socially engaged with Family and Friends until the last year. Quite suddenly, she seemed to undergo dramatic changes in activities and personality. She lost her balance and bearing within her own home and fell several times. After being taken to the emergency room, they discovered that she had suffered a series of strokes. She experienced some numbness on her right side. She was eventually transferred to a Skilled Nursing Facility. She seemed to cognitively disengage completely from her surroundings. She appeared to talk to people not present. She tried to eat non-food items. She repeatedly talked about catching a train. She no longer recognized Family Members. While in the SNF she suffered another stroke and contracted aspiration pneumonia. She did not respond well to IV antibiotics and as her strength and health continued to deteriorate, she was placed on Hospice Care.

As a Hospice Volunteer, sooner or later You will be asked to go on assignments where, in addition to other serious illnesses, Patients are suffering with various degrees of cognitive decline. Each of the above three cases are unique examples of the types of conditions and situations that You may encounter. Severe cognitive deficits during End-of-Life situations can make caregiving enormously complicated for all parties. In these cases, specialized strategies and approaches are needed in order to effect meaningful interactions with Patients and Loved Ones.

Similar to all other Hospice assignments, your preliminary work is critical. You need to try to compile as complete a profile of the Patient's medical, psychological, social, functional, and cognitive conditions as possible. If the Patient has a history or diagnosis of severe cognitive problems, an in-depth and thorough discussion of these issues is essential to the Volunteer prior to the initial visit. In these cases, the assigned Social Worker might be able to provide a valuable perspective on the Patient and surrounding Loved Ones.

Again, during your preparatory questions, it will be helpful if You think in terms of the cognitive "dimensions" described above. This is to say, do Patients suffer any memory lapses? Do they appear confused or disengaged from their surroundings? Do they exhibit hallucinatory engagements? Do they lack any sense of future plans or events? Are they at all capable of grasping new information? Do they have the ability to understand and also speak verbal communication? Do they have any extreme behavioral problems? Having basic answers to and insights from these questions will aid You tremendously on your first visit. This information will also serve as a baseline of Patient assessments during subsequent visits.

In order to be effective as a Hospice or Palliative Care Volunteer, You will need to develop some very specialized "interpersonal skills" when dealing with Patients suffering with various cognitive deficits. As always, your basic objective in spending time with Patients is to maintain or enhance their present Quality-of-Life. When dealing with very sick people who are also struggling with cognitive problems, your approach needs to be tailored to their specific cognitive "reality". Again, every Individual is unique and there can be enormous variations among Patients with cognitive issues. There are however, some very generalized and yet effective ways in which to interact with People suffering cognitive limitations.

These principles and practices are well known to healthcare professionals who deal with such Patients on a daily basis. These practical strategies include the following attitudes and approaches.

- As with all Hospice or Palliative encounters, You should go into a visit with a "neutral energy and assumptions" perspective. Then try to get a feel for the current attitudes and moods of the Patient and other Individuals present. Sometimes, this is more difficult when dealing with Patients with cognitive issues.

- However, when approaching and all during your time with the Patient, You should try to maintain an easy-going, friendly, smiling, gentle demeanor. This should help to dispel any reaction on the part of the Patient that You are seen as somehow a "threat" to be feared.

- If some degree of verbal communication is possible, make easy and brief eye contact intermittently. Always try to face the Patient directly when speaking.

- Always speak slowly and clearly. Repeat or rephrase questions or comments in an even cadence as necessary. However, try to avoid sounding condescending as if you are treating the Patient like a child.

- At the start of each visit, introduce yourself using your first name only. Do not be concerned if the Patient does not know or remember You. You might show them your printed name on your nametag. (Avoid this if You decide the word "Hospice" or "Palliative" that appears on your nametag might upset the Patient?) Tell the Patient that You are there just to spend a little time as a friendly visitor.

- Always practice so-called *"Validation Therapy"*. This means that when a Patient appears to be dealing with distorted perceptions, or hallucinations, or with irrational emotional pain, You should never try to resolve or correct or explain away the ideas or realities that the Individual is grappling with. Doing so is never really successful and can foster far more suffering in the Patient. As a visitor, You should simply endeavor to "go along with whatever the Patient is claiming". For example, a Patient might state that her husband will be in to visit her and You know for certain that her husband died two years ago. You should never try to correct her or explain to her that her husband is dead and will not be in to see her. Within her private present-day cognitive world, she may suddenly experience the terrible grief and sorrow of losing her husband for the first time. Obviously, this serves no meaningful purpose. Instead, as a visitor You should go along with her story and say that when You see him, You will tell him where his wife is. You try to "validate" whatever the Patient's reality is currently.

* If the Patient asks You the same question over and over, ("looping") You should simply repeat the answer over and over. Do not say that You have already answered that question nor ask why the Patient does not recall your answer from before.

* Patients may or may not "enjoy" holding your hand during the visit.

* Some Patients may seem to respond to soft music or to looking at bright picture-images. These pictures might include images of animals, nature scenes, babies, or children. They might include pictures of things that the Person identified with over a lifetime, such as gardens or trains or the military.

* Some Patients may retain some capacity to still enjoy puzzles or arts and crafts, drawing or painting.

* Sometimes during visits, Patients may be mumbling, disengaged, incoherent, "off in another world" or semi-conscious. Sometimes the most meaningful activity is for You to simply bring a quiet, calm compassionate presence to the Patient and surroundings.

The above suggestions should help You cultivate a peaceful and sincere encounter with a Patient with extraordinary challenges. It has been stated that even during the advanced stages of progressive dementia, it seems there is still an "emotional being" underlying the chaos and the terrible sense of a vanishing selfhood. As a Hospice or Palliative Care Volunteer, it might be said that You are striving to still somehow connect with that emotional level.

CHAPTER 17

THE PATIENT FACING DYING AND DEATH

▲ ▲ ▲

As A HOSPICE VOLUNTEER, IT is important for You to constantly keep in mind that every Human Being's End-of-Life journey is unique. This means that your Volunteer experiences with each Patient will also be unique. The course or trajectory of each Individual's gradual decline up to the finality of death will vary tremendously. Different individuals respond to medical and psychological strategies differently. Likewise, People react to intense personal and existential challenges very differently. This differentiation varies widely from those Individuals that are eventually referred to a Hospice status as compared to those Individuals who die suddenly or unexpectedly. Again, as a Volunteer, You may visit a Patient once or You may visit many times over the course of many months.

However, there are a variety of common *"psychological states or moods"*, *"behavioral activities or actions"*, and *"physical conditions and changes"* that Individuals facing dying and death "might" experience. Patients struggling within End-of-Life situations may exhibit one or some or many of these Human patterns. Again, every Person's dying trajectory is unique. However, as a Hospice Volunteer, it can be enormously helpful to You when working with Patients to have some understanding of these various factors. When You first encounter many of these conditions and changes, You might be uneasy or even shocked by what You witness. You will quickly learn to accept these issues as an integral part of the Human dying experience. Again, the Hospice approach does not seek to slow down nor hasten the natural biological process of dying. Over time, You will learn to recognize many of these issues and thereby be better able to engage the Patient in meaningful ways. As always, You are not there to "resolve" their psychological or behavioral or physical difficulties. You are there to offer a compassionate, patient, and empathic Human presence during their challenging journey.

Elizabeth Kubler-Ross

One of the most significant pioneering works into researching the personal experiences of Humans confronting dying and death was conducted by the Psychiatrist Elizabeth Kubler-Ross. Her assessments and conclusions were first published in 1969 in her groundbreaking book *"On Death & Dying"*. She summarized her findings after interviewing scores of terminally ill Patients and their close Loved Ones over almost three years. Her research has had a lasting and profound effect on how many Physicians now deal with their terminally ill Patients. Her research also helped pave the way for the development and implementation of the practical ideals within the Hospice and Palliative Care movements.

Kuber-Ross originally developed a "five-stage" model to describe the mental and emotional experiences Individuals often report when struggling with the inevitability of impending death. She detailed these five issues as follows.

1. *Denial:* This is the first and most common emotional response to the initial news of being given a formal medical diagnosis of a terminal disease. It often consists of a sudden and intense shock of disbelief about such news. It may include mind-numbing fear, confusion and a basic refusal to accept the reality of such information. Often the first response is some form of subtle denial which can take many forms. Patients and Loved Ones may "hope" that the Doctor's initial diagnoses and lab results are somehow wrong. They often seek out a second or third medical opinion or assessment. They often cling to the possibility of finding some

high-tech medical intervention and eventual cure. They hope that the Patient is a statistical anomaly and will somehow recover, in spite of the terminal diagnosis. Ultimately they may believe that a spiritual miracle healing might take place.

2. *Anger:* This powerful and agitated reaction can also take many forms. The Patient, as well as surrounding Loved Ones may feel a terrible sense of somehow being a "victim". Anger may be directed towards the disease itself, towards the medical profession for "failing" the Patient, towards God for allowing such a disease and even towards oneself for "causing" the illness. The terrible questions asked by the Patient are often *"Why me?" and "Why now?"*

3. *Bargaining:* This describes when the Patient or Loved One tries to "negotiate" a deal or agreement with God or Angels or Spiritual Beings to circumvent the disease. This is usually done in private by the Patient or Loved One. Patients may propose a "win-win" situation. Examples might be such as, "If You will heal me, I promise to thereafter do good works"; "If you will let me live long enough to see my Child graduate from college, then I will donate money to the college."

4. *Depression:* This entails profound sadness or sorrow in reacting to the progression of the disease and the inexorable march towards impending death. It usually stems from a sense of hopelessness with the realization that everything that is joyful and meaningful in life will soon end. This depression can have a clinical or situational basis.

5. *Acceptance:* This is the final surrendering to the inevitability of one's own death. This is not to be understood necessarily as a happy or contented stage. It is acceptance of an absolute finality. It may entail a calm and genuine recognition of an existential reality. It may include an apathetic detachment and withdrawal from one's surroundings. Dying People tend to become progressively less aware of and less engaged in the physical world around them.

Since 1975 several other researchers have developed and expanded a variety of different interpretations of the original work of Kubler-Ross. They have recognized the internal validity of her "stages" model, but have suggested that a strict progression from one stage into another may not be entirely accurate. An Individual suffering a terminal disease may move in and out or even back and forth among these stages. Many Patients seem to experience multiple stages at the same time, such as *Denial and Depression*. Still others may remain entrenched in a single stage and never get passed it, such as *Bargaining* or *Anger*.

Again, every End-of-Life journey is unique. The Human reality is that when Individuals receive and accept a terminal diagnosis, their entire "world-orientation" undergoes a sudden and dramatic change. Everything they focus on, everything they value, everything they hope for or cherish is permanently compromised or altered.

In addition to the five "stages" described above, as a Hospice Volunteer, You will encounter a vast and complex array of other "*psychological, behavioral and physical factors*" that Patients may exhibit. During the courses of your visitations with them, they may show one or more of the following aspects in reacting to their declining conditions.

Psychological States or Moods

* *Anxiety, Fear, Dread:* This is a natural Human response to the confusion of not knowing exactly how a terminal illness will progress. This includes the uncertainty of not knowing how long the rest of life will be. It usually includes *anxiety* over the anticipation of physical and cognitive pain and incapacity. It may encompass *fear* over ending up on a ventilator, being tube fed, mentally confused or in diapers. It often fosters *dread* over the absolute ending of life and the finality of death.
* *Sorrow, Grief:* This is the common reaction to the inevitable series of Human "losses" associated with dying and death; includes

the "anticipation" of losing one's identity, losing loving relationships, capacity for work, value to others, opportunity to engage in life, etc.

* *Bewilderment:* This often develops with Patients feeling compelled to ask sweeping questions, such as "How and why could this happen?" or "What higher purpose could possibly be served by suffering and death?" or "How could a loving God allow such terrible things to occur?" Enduring dying and inevitable death sometimes fosters a feeling of injustice or unfairness in a Patient.

* *Shortened or Vanishing "Time-Line":* This describes the emotional perception that a normal Human perspective on upcoming events has become meaningless. Hospice and Palliative Care Patients' experiential "time-line" tends to shrink dramatically or disappear completely. Planning or anticipating future situations becomes inherently uncertain and problematic. They may admit to such limitations by saying "I probably won't make it to Christmas!" or "Who knows if I'll be around then!"

* *Reminiscence:* This usually manifests as a powerful urge to reflect back over the significant events and important relationships with People over the Patient's life. Individuals facing End-of-Life situations often feel compelled to review, to evaluate and to judge their decisions and experiences during their Life Course. These can encompass issues of great excitement and joy as well as great sorrow and regret.

* *Situational Needs:* This develops sometimes when Patients express concerns about the impact their disease and dying will have on Family and Loved Ones. They often express anxiety over the financial state of affairs they are leaving behind. They may talk about the high cost of their disease and feeling powerless to change the situation. They may feel compelled to give instructions about their household, possessions, pets, etc. They may talk about their anxiety concerning how Family Members will get

along when the Patient is finally gone. They may even offer guidance on their own funerals or memorial services.

* *Relationship Needs:* As the end of a Human Life draws near, most Patients become more focused on the relationships they have had with specific "Persons" in their life. The primary importance of People tends to supersede any on-going interest in "things". They may express a powerful need to see certain Loved Ones. They may want to simply tell them they love them and to say a last good-bye. Some Patients may suddenly feel a terrible need for closure or reconciliation with a certain Family Member from which they have suffered a past estrangement.

* *Religious or Spiritual Needs:* This describes the powerful need many Patients feel as they perceive the end of their lives drawing to a close. Many Humans believe that the "meaningfulness" of their life is grounded within a spiritual or transcendental reality. Many Individuals will engage in an intense reexamination of their traditional religious beliefs and upbringing. They may request visitations and council with respected religious Leaders. Still others may seek out a new and wider range of religious or spiritual ideas.

* *Loss of Interests:* This encompasses the gradual decrease in wanting to engage in activities and events that Patients normally did in the past. These Individuals often become withdrawn from or disinterested in routine pleasurable hobbies or interests. As a terminal disease progresses, they sometimes seem to prefer solitude and inactivity.

* *"Confusion or Disorientation":* This deals with the common experience of Patients with advanced serious illness becoming disengaged from "normal reality". They sometimes tend to lose "orientation" to people, place, time and situation (See the Chapter on Cognitive Issues in End-of-Life Care). They may start talking about needing to pack belongings for a trip. They may express an urgency about catching a plane or a train. They may begin

to talk in a "matter-of-fact" way to "unseen Persons", including long-dead Relatives. They may start to describe the presence of Angels or images of Heaven.

BEHAVIORAL ACTIVITIES OR ACTIONS

Again, in addition to the variety of psychological issues described above, Hospice and Palliative Care Patients may exhibit one or more of the following "behaviors" intermittently over the course of their gradual decline.

* *Difficulties with ADLs:* This refers to Patients becoming physically weaker and losing mobility and dexterity as their conditions worsen. They often become less able to perform simple "activities of daily living", such as eating, going to the bathroom, dressing, etc. They may need assistance with transferring from a bed into a wheelchair. They often require increasing levels of hands-on care as time goes on.

* *Sleeping more:* This deals with a very common behavioral pattern as Individuals become sicker over time. They tend to sleep more and more. This often includes sleeping more during the daylight hours. As death draws nearer, Patients sometimes appear to sleep almost continuously.

* *Social Withdrawal:* This describes the gradual decline in wanting to engage in normal social encounters with Friends and even some Family Members. As Patients become less interested in the surrounding physical environment, they may also become less interested in social activities. As they become weaker, social interactions might turn into an exhausting burden which they simply prefer to avoid.

* *Agitation and Restlessness:* This refers to the difficult behaviors of Patients seeming to become anxious or "out of sorts" with their situation. These behaviors may reflect underlying

emotional stressors such as anger or confusion or depression. Patients may sometimes jump out of bed and try to leave the room. They may toss and turn and finally fall out of bed. They might appear stressed out and distracted from their immediate surroundings.

* *Changes in Eating and Drinking:* This deals with the very complex patterns of Individuals taking in food and hydration over the course of dying and death. As their conditions worsen, Patients will often begin to take in significantly less food and liquids. They might claim that they do not feel like eating, that they have no appetite or that food is making them feel sick. As they draw near to death, many Patients simply refuse to eat or even drink anything. These behaviors often cause Family and Loved Ones great concern. However, professionals who work with dying Individuals report that these "extreme" behaviors are quite common and should be respected and accepted.

* *"Death-Bed Visions":* As mentioned elsewhere, Patients sometimes begin to describe "other-worldly" perceptions. As they get closer to the event of death, they may begin talking to "Persons not physically present". They may claim to be conversing with a dead Loved One or with a guardian Angel or a religious Figure. They might describe celestial landscapes or cathedrals. Family Members and medical Professionals often dismiss these behaviors as caused by hallucinations or confusion.

PHYSICAL CONDITIONS AND CHANGES

Similar to the basic descriptions of the various *psychological* and *behavioral* issues detailed above, there can be a complex array of *"physical conditions and changes"* that may be displayed by Patients struggling within a dying trajectory. Again, not every Patient will exhibit every condition. Sometimes a specific physical symptom will manifest for a short time only.

These possible physical manifestations do not emerge in any set pattern or progression. They may vary a great deal in terms of severity and duration. Some of these are as follows.

- *Weakness, Fatigue (Asthenia):* This describes Patients' gradual loss of physical muscular strength and balance. It includes an overall weakness that can prevent Patients from performing routine common activities. As Individuals draw nearer to death, they often become so weak as to remain bedridden.
- *Weight Loss (Cachexia):* This is the gradual wasting away of basic body composition, including muscle mass, fat stores and even major organ structures.
- *Physical Pain:* Terminal diseases often cause progressive types of pain in various locations within the body. This discomfort can take many forms such as generalized or localized, aching, dull, sharp, intermittent or continuous. Such pain is a "subjective experience" of the Patient and must be verbally reported or recognized behaviorally by Caregivers. Effective "pain management" is a primary objective in Hospice and Palliative Care.
- *Sleep Disturbance:* This often occurs when a Patient's normal sleep patterns become disrupted. They often become restless, sleep less during the night and more during daylight hours. As a terminal disease worsens, Patients usually sleep more and more. As death approaches, they often drift in and out of consciousness (sleep) most of the time. Medications administered to alleviate pain and anxiety may also contribute to this behavior.
- *Lessened Food and Fluid Intake:* As a life ending disease progresses, the Patient will often gradually want to consume less food and fluids. This will contribute to Cachexia (wasting away). Towards the end of life, they will often begin to refuse any food or liquids. This can be especially disturbing to Loved Ones, but

is a natural process for many at the End-of-Life. (See *Changes in Eating and Drinking* above)

* *Difficulties with Bladder and Bowel Function:* These issues can take many forms, such as incontinence, constipation, diarrhea, infections, bloating, etc. Effectively managing these factors are among the most difficult challenges both Patients and Family Caregivers will face.

* *Nausea and Vomiting:* With the dramatic changes that often occur to the digestive tract during a terminal disease, some Patients suffer severe bouts of nausea and vomiting. This can lead to pain and discomfort in the throat, malnutrition and dehydration. These ailments usually require professional medical interventions such as medications or even IV support.

As always, the overarching goals in Hospice and Palliative Care are to foster "comfort care" and the highest possible Quality-of-Life during the final stages of Human life. These goals encompass addressing each of the *phycological, behavioral,* and *physical issues* described above. Of course, not every Patient will experience or display each of these factors during the course of their decline and dying. Every Human dying trajectory is unique. The treatment and support for each Individual will be tailored to that specific Person. Likewise, the Volunteer's engagement and interactions with each Patient will vary.

AT THE THRESHOLD OF DEATH

Again, every Human passing away is different. People who die suddenly due to an unexpected event such as an accident or heart attack generally do not end up in Hospice or Palliative Care. Patients who have been taken under Hospice or Palliative Care are usually enduring a drawn out or long-term disease course. Most of these Individuals will experience at least some of the conditions and processes described above over a period of weeks or months. <u>It is virtually impossible to accurately predict the actual day and time that final death will occur.</u> However, there are several factors that may be observed as Patients draw nearer to death. Some of these are a more severe form of the issues detailed above. Hospice and Palliative Care Caregivers will sometimes use the phrase *"actively dying"* when describing the situation in which death is thought to be *"imminent"*. These factors might include the following.

* *Fluctuations in Blood Pressure and Pulse Rate:* These factors can vary up and down dramatically as the Patient nears death. If the Individual is in a home setting or in a regular hospital bed, these fluctuations might generally go unnoticed. As the Patient gets close to dying, blood pressure and pulse rate will tend to decrease.

* *Swallowing Problems (Dysphagia):* Towards the end, if the Person is still taking in some nutrition or fluids orally, they may experience some aggravation with swallowing. They may even ingest material into the lungs which can cause serious problems, such as pneumonia or other respiratory infections.

* *Refusal to take Food or Fluids:* Oftentimes, as the very end draws near, the Patient will simply refuse any further food or liquids. The assumption is that the process of active digestion has essentially shut down and it is a physical and psychological burden to ingest any further substances.

* *Bluishness or Cold in Extremities:* Sometimes the Patient's feet, legs, hands and arms will begin to feel cold to the touch and take on a bluish coloration. This is generally due to poor circulation to these parts of the body, which may be caused by the diminishing strength of the pumping heart.

* *Lessening of Bladder and Bowel Activity:* Urination and bowel output will often slow down and even stop in the final days and hours. Again, the entire digestive tract as well as metabolic processes are slowed or even shutting down.

* *Changes in Breathing:* This is a very common behavior and can be recognized by anyone closely observing the Patient. Breathing patterns may become strained, shallow, disrupted and uneven. The Person may appear to stop actually breathing for a short period of time and then begin again. Sometimes it is very difficult to even tell if the Patient is breathing.

* *Continuous Sleeping or Unconsciousness:* In Hospice and Palliative Care, it is very common for dying Patients to sleep or be unconscious most of the time. Sometimes this may be associated with medications being given to manage pain or stress. However, this pattern is very common to all Individuals during the final phase of life, and should be regarded as an integral part of the natural dying process.

Again, all the varied and complex issues described above *"may"* be a part of a Patient's enduring the End-of-Life experience. As a Hospice Volunteer, You will encounter each and every one of these scenarios at some point in your work. They should all be understood as part of the Human experience of dying and death.

DEATH IN HOSPICE

As a Hospice Volunteer, You will usually not be present when a Patient You are regularly visiting actually dies. This is simply because You normally spend only one or two hours per week with that Person. However, if You work in this field long enough, You may well be there at the point of death. There is an increased possibility of this if You work as a Vigil Volunteer. (See the Chapter on Vigil Support)

In general, the People who are referred into Hospice Care are in the end stages of a long-term, serious disease trajectory. Oftentimes with elderly Individuals, these diseases are some form of chronic conditions that have turned acute over time. For example, a Person may have been suffering for years with congestive heart failure (CHF), chronic obstructive pulmonary disease (COPD), diabetes, kidney disease, Parkinson's, Alzheimer's and other types of dementia, etc. Many People even struggle with certain forms of cancer over months or even years. These are the types of medical situations in which Hospice or Palliative Care Support has a chance of being effective. Individuals who die suddenly or unexpectedly as in an accident or when a lethal disease was not properly recognized or diagnosed will not end up in Hospice or Palliative Care.

Within a Hospice or Palliative Care setting, the actual event of death is usually a subtle and calm passing away. Sometimes, the exact point of dying is difficult to discern. Breathing gradually becomes quiet and shallow. The Individual may even appear to stop breathing for several seconds and then resume respiration. The vast majority of Hospice and Palliative Care Patients will usually die while asleep or "unconscious". The reality is that most of these People appear to die at ease and peacefully.

ACTIVITIES

▲ ▲ ▲

"The most profound realization that dying Human
Beings reveal is that People matter – things don't!"

COL

*"People may disagree about what quality of life
is worth sustaining and there is far from a social
consensus. But for each individual, it is relevant
to consider what quality of life the person, himself
or herself, would consider worth sustaining."*

IRA BYOCK

*"Compassion asks us to go where it hurts, to enter
into the places of pain, to share in brokenness,
fear, pain and anguish. Compassion challenges
us to cry out with those in misery, to mourn with
those who are lonely...Compassion means full
immersion in the condition of being human."*

HENRI J.M. NOUWEN

HELEN

▲ ▲ ▲

I WAS READY AND LOOKING for my next assignment with Vitas Innovative Hospice. By then, I had worked as a Volunteer in Hospice support for several years with multiple Agencies. I had also worked in the Social Services department in two different Skilled Nursing Facilities. I was generally confident about working with any Hospice Patient with any medical or cognitive conditions in any "home setting". I called and talked directly to the Volunteer Coordinator about possible assignments. I requested that she give me the most challenging Patient possible that had not yet been given to the Volunteer pool. She asked me if I would be willing to begin visitations with "Helen" who was living in a large Skilled Nursing Facility on a permanent "custodial" basis. She was an 85 year old widower. Helen's medical history included treatment for "Alzheimer's". Her primary medical diagnosis was "cerebral atherosclerosis" and her secondary diagnosis was "cerebrovascular disease, unspecified". Over the past several months, she had apparently displayed many episodes of temporary confusion and disorientation. I understood going in that this would be a very challenging assignment.

When I first met Helen, she was effectively bedridden. She shared a room with another woman, but that roommate was rarely there when I visited. During our first encounter, Helen appeared somewhat "alert and oriented" to her surroundings and to my presence. She was able to respond to simple questions about where and when she was born, her Husband, work, Children and Grandchildren, etc. However, during the course of our conversation, she would intermittently become distracted and agitated saying "Father in Heaven help me, I am not safe here". She would then seem to quickly calm down and resume talking directly to me. Given her diagnoses and in that I had spent time working within the Dementia Ward in Skilled Nursing, Helen's behaviors did not surprise nor concern me. I tried to engage her in conversation as much as possible. I also played soft and melodic music on my iphone which she seemed to respond to in a positive manner. She would listen to the music and grow more calm. She would then appear to doze off periodically. This first visit only lasted about 35 minutes.

During subsequent visits, Helen was sometimes engaged and coherent. She would respond to simple, immediate questions, such as "Are you hungry?" or "Are you warm enough?". She could also respond to more abstract questions, such as "What state were you born in?" or "What year were you born in?'. At times, she displayed no "religious ramblings" while at other times she appeared preoccupied with such topics. During one visit, she kept repeating the phrase "Jesus help me" and "Oh Lord help me". She even appeared to address me as Jesus. When I gently said that I was leaving, she became anxious and said "No – Jesus, you can't leave me now". So, I sat down next to her bed until she seemed to settle down.

Also, during a couple of my visits, I found her sound asleep. As per my routine, I gently called her name to see if she might respond. In general, she did not. She appeared to be calm and breathing regularly, so I simply left her alone. I sat quietly by her side for about 30-45 minutes.

My visits with Helen went on for about seven weeks. I never ran into any of her Family Members. Our time together was spent with Her, me and sometimes "Jesus". As a Hospice Volunteer, You are there to try to engage that Patient in whatever is most meaningful at the moment. The Patient should dictate the pace, duration, activities and content of each visit.

Then I received a phone call from the Agency informing me that Helen has passed quietly in the middle of the night. There were not a lot of details about her last days and moments on earth, but hopefully she is now with Jesus and the Lord!

CHAPTER 18

Suggested Activities During
a Friendly Visit

▲ ▲ ▲

THE FOLLOWING IS A LIST of possible *"Activities"* that the Hospice Volunteer might choose from to engage the Patient during a friendly visitation. This is only a "partial" set of suggestions. There may well be many other types of activities that the Volunteer might develop for specific Patients. Again, as each Patient's situation is unique, so too is each individual visit. <u>As always, the type and complexity and duration of these activities will depend on the current physical, emotional and cognitive conditions of the Patient. The overall objective of each of these various activities is ideally for social interaction, for mental or emotional enhancement and for energetic and fun stimulation.</u>

Prior to the initial visit, the Volunteer will generally receive some guidance during the discussion with the Agency Coordinator about potential activities to introduce with the Patient. The admitting Nurse or Social Worker will have usually compiled information to be included in the case file about the Family, work career, hobbies and interests of the Patient. Such factors will help to guide the types of activities chosen for each visit.

The interactions with the Patient may be affected by the "home setting" within which visitations take place. As mentioned, visiting a Hospice Patient living in a private residence will be different from visiting one living in a facility of some kind. The first visit is usually spent with the Volunteer, Patient and any Loved Ones present introducing themselves and just getting to know each other. During this encounter, there is usually some discussion about what the Patient might be interested in doing during on-going visitations. From all these elements, a tentative plan for activities can be developed.

The Volunteer should always have specific activities in mind when going into each visitation. The guiding principle should always be to strive to engage the Patient in whatever activities that Patient will find most meaningful at the time. However, Hospice Volunteers should always be flexible and ready to adapt to whatever situation they may walk into. (Recall the *"neutral emotion-energy assumption"* the Volunteer should adopt before each new or next visit.) Sometimes, the Patient's physical, emotional and cognitive status are similar with the previous visit. Sometimes they are radically different from the prior visit. The Volunteer may need to completely change the plans for the current encounter. The following list offers some guidelines about possible Activities.

SUGGESTED ACTIVITIES

* Ask about and discuss the Patient's routine events of the present day so far; sleep, meals, comfort level, activities. (Key questions: "How are You doing today?" "How are You doing this afternoon?")
* Discuss the various experiences and events since You last visited the Patient. ("How have You been *over the past few days, since we last met?*" "*Have You had any visitors – any Family Members or Friends?*" "*How have You been sleeping?*' "*What have You been eating?*", *etc.)*
* Discuss specific topics that You as a Volunteer know the Patient has a long-term interest in, such as a chosen hobby, career path and interests, activities such as camping, sailing, military service, civic groups, etc.
* Explore lifetime "Biographical Themes". These can take many forms such as informal, random questions or highly structured

"Life Review" or "Guided Autobiography". (See the expanded Section listing specific Biographical Topics and Questions)

- Talk about the Patients' cherished Family Members, close Loved Ones and Friends that have been and remain important in the Patient's life.
- Go through a Photo Album and discuss the events and memories evoked by this personal record.
- Review and discuss important personal pictures and memorabilia around the room or home.
- Engage in so-called "word games" such as "unscramble letters", "match meanings", "trivia questions", "word circle and crossword puzzles", "finish the clichés", etc.
- Read aloud writings that are meaningful to the Patient, such as Bible passages, favorite stories or poems, etc.
- Discuss current news stories and events.
- Play simple or more complex card or board games.
- Arrange to be able to listen to some music of the type, genre and hits that the Patient has enjoyed over a lifetime, such as "Gospel", "Big Band", "Folk", "Rock and Roll", etc.
- Engage in various Arts and Crafts or Hobby projects.
- Watch favorite television shows.
- Watch a favorite old movie (DVD).
- Watch old Family home movies if available and discuss events and People involved.
- Accompany Patient on walking trip (using wheelchair as necessary) outside to garden or park (as permitted by the Agency).
- Take Patient on a ride in your car (as permitted by your Agency).
- <u>Or, sit quietly, say and do nothing other than offering your caring and compassionate presence.</u>

As a rule, the Patient will be more able and interested in more complex activities during your early visits than in your later visits. Again, the Patient's mood and conditions are the ultimate factors guiding the course of each visit.

CHAPTER 19

REMINISCINDING ACTIVITIES

▲ ▲ ▲

IT MAY WELL BE THAT the most meaningful and powerful "activity" that the Hospice Volunteer engages in with a Patient is _"reminiscing" about that Patient's life._

When Individuals are suddenly confronted with the specter of their own impending mortality, they often respond with a heightened sense of urgency to "look back" over their lives. This might include reflecting back over the stages of One's life, or reliving memories, or thinking and feeling about the patterns of various experiences. It may include pondering over pivotal events, People, interests and passions that have comprised that Person's life. Such reminiscence may take the form of discussions with others or it may be the private remembering of events in a Person's life through daydreaming, or nostalgia. It may encompass not only simple recall, but reflection, assessment and interpretation of One's life course, choices, valuations and assumptions about the life as lived. This will quite naturally include memories that are both joyful and painful.

It has been said that an Individual's life is best understood as a personal narrative of a series of "stories". To recount a Person's biography is to describe that life as a story. As with all Human Beings, that Person's private story intersects with Others' life stories and must be understood within the wider arena of still other social and cultural stories. The overall meaning of these various stories can be categorized as historical (factual) or metaphorical (existential). The Patient will determine within which category each story belongs. In Hospice support, reminiscence is the process of recounting One's personal stories.

As a Hospice Volunteer, You will almost always find that Patients are very interested in discussing the events and memories they have about their lives. This will often take up the majority of the time You spend with them from one visit to the next. The more experience You have, the better You will become at respectfully posing simple questions and drawing out personal responses from Patients about their life stories. Initially, You may have to have a series of questions and ideas written down when approaching a Patient on a first visit or even during subsequent visits. As You become more comfortable and familiar with the process, You will be able to formulate questions from memory.

Obviously, in order to be effective, when engaging a Patient in life reminiscing, that Patient will have to retain a significant level of cognitive capacity. This encompasses basic memory, orientation, communication and understanding. When trying to prompt such Patients into talking openly about their life stories, the questions should be asked in a calm, friendly conversational manner. You should never come across as firing a bunch of questions at the Patient. Ask the questions and then let the Person run with them. Some Individuals are more talkative than others. The length and depth of responses should always be determined by what the Patient appears to be comfortable with. Always let the Patient control and drive the narrative. The Volunteer's role is simply to prompt or facilitate the Patient's reminiscing about life events. It is important for You to remember that You are not there as a Therapist. You are not there to interpret or explain or reframe or assess the Patient's stories. You are there as an empathic listener only. You are there as a kind, compassionate friendly companion.

The following is a list of suggested questions You might use as a Friendly Visitor. These are specific questions You ask the Patient directly. They do not need to be asked in any specific order. Oftentimes, a single question will lead to lengthy answers and associated memories that take up the entire visit. Other responses may only take a minute or two. Again, friendly conversation is the guideline and ideal.

- "Where were You born? Where did You grow up? Did You move many times when You were a child?
- Where did You go to school? Did You have a favorite subject of study? Did You do extra-curricular activities – art, theater, science, sports, etc. Did You attend college? What did You study?
- Did You or any Family Member have any significant health issues when You were young?
- Tell me about Your Parents, Grandparents. What kind of work did Your Dad do? Your Mother? Did she work outside the house?
- Tell me about your brothers and sisters – growing up.
- Are any / all of these people still with us? Are You still close to any / all of them?
- Tell me about your current Significant Other, your Spouse or Partner (if appropriate). If You don't mind my asking, have You been married before this Person came into your life? Can You remember the very first time You saw and met your Spouse or Partner? How long have You two been together?
- Tell me about your Children (any and all "Children" as appropriate). When and where were they born? What was it like raising them? What special interests did they have growing up? Where are they now and what are they up to? Do You get to see them very much?
- Do You have any Grandchildren / Greatgrandchildren? Where are they living? Do You get to see them much?
- Tell me about your "war stories" if appropriate. (WWII, Korea, Vietnam, etc.) If You were not actively engaged in the war, what did You and your Family do during this period?
- What kind of work / career did You have? Did You have more than one career? Did You work in more than one industry or profession or trade? Did You work outside the home?

- Do You belong to any formal Religion? Is this helpful to You now? Is this still important to You? Would You say that You are spiritual but not religious?
- As an adult, how many times did You move over the years? What different states and parts of the country have You lived in? Do You still have a favorite place?
- Over the years, did You develop any special hobbies, activities or interests? Are You still able to enjoy any of these now?
- Where have You traveled over the years? Did You ever go outside this country? Do You have a favorite place outside the continental United States? When was the last time You visited there?
- (If retired) What kinds of activities have You been involved with since You retired? Are You still able to enjoy some of these?
- As You look back over your life, is there any specific activity You would still like to engage in? Do You think we might be able to do it a little?

Again, this is only a partial list of questions You might try to engage the Patient in reminiscing about a "life story". These basic questions may well lead to many other areas of discussion. They may lead to bringing out an old photo album or old home movies packed with Family memories. They might point to pictures and memorabilia on the walls. As mentioned, older People (like the vast majority of Hospice Patients) dwell and find deep purpose and meaning within their memories. This is the pool of experience and emotions You are tapping into with life review.

FRIENDLY VISITOR

▲ ▲ ▲

"FREQUENTLY ASKED QUESTIONS"

* **How do I find out about Hospice Agencies and opportunities in my area?**
    * The best and most practical way is to search the internet for specific websites of Hospice Agencies near You. You might be surprised at how many Agencies there are. You may also find listings for organizations that offer Hospice Care as well as "Home Health Care", "Adult Day Care", "Assisted Living", etc. Focus on any websites that list "Hospice" as part of their operation.
* **What is the best way to approach an Agency about Volunteer opportunities near me?**
    * The simplest way is to call the Agency and ask to speak to the "Volunteer Coordinator". That Person will be happy to talk to You over the phone and will usually ask to schedule an appointment to meet You face-to-face. Remember, according to Medicare directives, the Agency is required to continually recruit and develop Volunteer resources.
* **Do I have to go through formal Training before I can begin work as a Volunteer?**
    * Medicare Regulations require all Hospice Volunteers to receive appropriate Training when entering this field. Most

Agencies have regularly scheduled Training sessions during a calendar year. Sometimes You may have to wait for weeks or even months to be enrolled in the next Training course. However, since the specific Medicare guidelines concerning Training allow for some leeway, your Agency may train You on an Individual basis to get You started. Check with your Coordinator about this possibility.

- **Do I really have to have a TB test, flu shot, MMR vaccinations, etc. before I can work as a Hospice Volunteer?**
  - Federal Medicare Regulations stipulate that Hospice Volunteers that interact directly with Patients must submit to a TB test. Beyond that, some Agencies may specify that additional clinical tests or precautions be taken by their Volunteers. This might include an annual flu shot or proof of current vaccinations status. As always, check with your particular Agency and You will generally have to comply with their policies.

- **Once I am fully trained and ready to go, how will I find out about new potential Volunteer Assignments with my Agency?**
  - There are several channels through which your Agency might put out this information. Coordinators will usually post a general list of open Assignments as a group email directed to all Volunteers. You can study through these and pick one that you might be interested in pursuing. Directly call the Coordinator to discuss the Case. At any time, You can call the Coordinator and ask about open Assignments. Also, sometimes the Coordinator may call You to offer a specific Assignment that the Agency feels You might have an affinity for.

- **Is it appropriate for me to request a specific type of Assignment; as e.g. to visit a Man or a Woman, a "home setting" as in a Private Home or an Assisted Living Facility, to work with a Patient with a unique background or specials interests, etc.?**

- Yes, You can certainly request a specific kind of Assignment and the Coordinator will generally try to match You up with such a Patient if available. If such an Assignment is not currently open, the Coordinator may look to match You up with such a Case if one presents itself.

- **Can the Agency "force" me or "require" me to take on a specific Assignment?**
  - Absolutely not; the Coordinator might try to gently persuade You to take an Assignment because You seem to be especially suited to that Patient. However, You are there on a voluntary basis and any reputable Agency will never try to force You to do anything.

- **Who is my primary contact at the Agency?**
  - In general, You will be communicating with the Volunteer Coordinator or the Coordinator's Assistant. However, You should always feel free to discuss important issues concerning a Patient Assignment with the Case Manager, the Social Worker, Spiritual Counselor, Home health Aide, etc. Just keep in mind that these Individuals are usually extremely busy working with many Cases at any given time. Be concise with your discussions and respectful of their time and obligations.

- **What is my relationship as a Volunteer to the Interdisciplinary Team or Group?**
  - Even though your Volunteer activity generally takes place away from the Agency offices, You are always considered to be an integral part of this Team or Group. You are free to discuss a Patient with them at any time. They will welcome your observations and interpretations about your experiences during your regular visits with the Patient. You are another "set of eyes" interacting directly with that Patient. Your timely Activity Logs provide critical real-time information about your visits.

- **Can I take on more than one Assignment at a time?**
  - Yes, if Assignments are available and You are capable of effectively working with more than one Patient at a time.
- **If I am anxious or uneasy about initially going on a challenging Assignment, can I have another seasoned Volunteer go with me; as e.g. going into a large complex facility?**
  - Yes, You can and should ask for Volunteer support through your Coordinator. When You take your first Assignment, the Agency will often require an experienced Volunteer go with You.
- **If for any reason, I am unable to continue with an on-going Assignment, can I quit?**
  - Yes, as a Volunteer, You can quit at any time. If for some reason You have trouble connecting with the Patient or Family Members, it might be better for everyone if You request a change in Assignments. Sometimes the Family may ask for a different Volunteer. Never take this personally. Loved Ones are struggling with an intense, chaotic and frightening time. Another Volunteer may somehow fit better on some emotional level with the Patient or Family.
- **How long do Assignments usually last?**
  - You may take an Assignment that lasts zero days; i.e. the Patient dies before your first visit. However, most Friendly Visitor Assignments usually span a period of several weeks up to several months. This is why You should consider each proposed Assignment carefully. It requires a serious and conscientious commitment to People coping with desperate and trying times.
- **How frequent should my visitations be with a Patient?**
  - In general, You will visit the Patient once or maybe twice each week. This is true whether You are going into a Private Home, an Assisted Living Facility or Skilled Nursing Facility.

- ***How should I plan my visitation schedule in each week?***
  - Always ask the Patient or Family Members during your initial contact with them if there is a best day and time for You to plan on visiting. In general, when going into a Private Home, it will be very important for You to visit at a regularly schedule time each week. The Patient and especially any Family Members present must be able to count on your showing up when expected. However, If You are going into a facility to visit a Patient, You may have more leeway as to when you actually visit. It may well be acceptable for You to visit in the "late morning" or "mid-afternoon" on any weekday.
- ***Should I call ahead before each visit?***
  - This will depend on what the Patient and Family requests. During your initial contact with the Family, You can ask them if they would prefer that you call before visiting. You can then ask them if they would prefer You to call ahead to confirm each subsequent visit. Some Families will prefer You to call, while others will not.
- ***What should I do if I am unable to visit a Patient on a given week?***
  - You should call the primary Family Member contact that You have interacted with before to inform that Person and to reschedule the next visit. You should also call or email the Coordinator about the situation.
- ***What should I do if I become sick prior to a visit?***
  - In general, if You are sick, it is best to never visit any Hospice Patient within any setting. Patient's usually have a compromised immune system and it is never a good idea to expose them to any potential infections.
- ***How important are my "Activity Logs" to the Agency?***
  - It is very important for You to fill these out and report them to your Agency in a timely manner. Any current and significant

"change in condition" of the Patient that You observe during your routine visit needs to be reported to the Coordinator right away. Such information may well be discussed at the regular meetings of the IDT or IDG. Also, according to Medicare Regulations, the Agency is required to document and keep on file, the minimum "5%" of hands-on care being provided by Volunteers. This calculation flows directly from your Activity Logs.

- ### What kind of personal records or files should I keep on Patients and visitations?
  - This is really up to You. As a Volunteer, You are not required to maintain such information. However, over time, You may find it useful to do so. The reality is that after You have seen a number of Patients, your memories of experiences with them will tend to "blur". You may want to be able to "compare" a Patient's changing conditions over time. You may want to refer back to Individual Patients and a private diary or confidential files will help You to do so.

- ### How important is "Patient Confidentiality" in my Volunteer work?
  - It is extremely important and will be an integral part of all your activities. Federal HIPAA Regulations are very stringent and Agencies can receive hefty fines for non-compliance. Your Training and Coordinator will educate You fully on the routine policies and procedures You must follow. This will affect any files You keep as well as any communications or correspondences You have with your Agency.

- ### Should I always wear my Hospice ID Badge during visits?
  - Generally, You should wear your ID Badge on all visitations. It is important for You to be readily identifiable as a member of the Hospice team wherever You go. When you go into a Private Residence, it will be helpful if Family Members see your badge and your name. It is especially important for You

to display your badge when going into a busy facility, so that all staff members will be able to readily identify whom You are. There may be one rare exception to this general practice. If Family Members tell You in private that they do not use the word "Hospice" around the Patient, You need to respect their wishes and put away your badge when visiting that Patient.

- **If asked by the Patient or Family Members, should I give them my private phone number, email address or home address?**
  - As a Volunteer, You should not give out such information. Gently tell the People You visit, that if they need to get ahold of You, they should call the Agency who will relay any message directly to You. It is important that professional "boundaries" be maintained as much as possible.

- **How long should each visitation last?**
  - Most of your visits will last one to two hours. Sometimes they may last longer depending on specific circumstances. However, the critical guiding principle should always be the interests and energy of the Patient. If that Patient appears to lose interest and grows tired or weary, You should look to gently end the visit. With this in mind, some visits may only last 30-45 minutes. On the other hand, if the Patient seems active, animated and enthused, your time there may go past the two hour window. This will be an on-going judgement call on your part with each visitation.

- **How long will "Respite" Assignments last?**
  - In general, these should also last one to two hours. Obviously, the exact time frame will be determined by how long the Family Member or Loved One is absent. Under some circumstances, this may stretch past the two hour limit. You should routinely confirm with the Person leaving for Respite how long they expect to be gone. As always, You will have essential phone contact information on Family Members in case You need to talk with them.

- *How long will "Vigil" Assignments last?*
  - These are specialized types of Assignments and usually have highly structured "time frames". These Assignments occur suddenly with the changing conditions of Individual Patients. The Coordinator will often post a new Vigil Assignment through a group email to trained Volunteers asking for Individuals to choose among a list of two hour time slots. The Coordinator's team may also call Volunteers to ask if they might be able to help. You may take a single "two hour stint" or you may take an afternoon slot from 2:00 to 4:00 until the Patient passes. The Coordinator will endeavor to fill all slots for as long as the Patient survives.
- *Will I be able or asked to perform routine "chores" for the Patient and Family, such as light housework, laundry, cleaning, cooking, etc.?*
  - Some Hospice Agencies offer these kinds of personal support, while others do not. It will depend on your Agency's individual practices and policies. If the Agency You work with does provide these forms of care, You will be offered the opportunity to engage in them. However, as always, You will never be forced to do so.
- *Will I be able or asked to do simple shopping for the Patient and Family, such as pick up groceries, drug store items or even prescription medications?*
  - Again, this will depend on your Agency's specific policies. Some offer these kinds of support, while others do not. Those that do will have paper procedures and forms designed to control expenditures and reimbursements as necessary. Picking up medications will require prior authorization and proper identification.
- *Will I be able or asked to take the Patient out in my personal car to run errands, go to medical appointments, go to the park, visit Friends, etc.*

- This depends on your Agency. Some will be set up to offer these services, while others will not. Taking a Patient out from their "home setting" requires very specific precautions. As an "employee" of the Agency, You could be held responsible (which means "legally liable") for events that could happen while the Patient is in your "charge". It could be a big problem if You were in a car accident, the Patient fell being transferred in and out of your car, or fell walking in a store, etc. Whether or not such support services are viable depends a great deal on the current functional and cognitive status of the Patient. Of course, the Agency would require current registration and insurance on any vehicle used. Given all these stringent limitations, this service can be enormously helpful to some Patients.

- **How should I respond if the Patient or any Family Member asks me specific "medical" or "legal" questions?**
  - You should reply by stating that, as a Volunteer, You cannot offer any formal opinions or interpretations on such matters. However, the Hospice Agency can certainly put the Patient or Family in touch with fully qualified Professionals that will be able to address such issues with them.

- **During regular visits, will I be asked to give "medications" to the Patient?**
  - During your brief regular visitation time, You should not be asked to administer any type of prescription or over-the-counter medications. This will be done routinely by Family or Hospice or facility Staff Caregivers.

- **During regular visits, will I be asked to "feed" the Patient?**
  - In general, as a Volunteer, You will never be asked to actually feed the Patient. This will be done by other qualified People.

- **During regular visits, am I allowed to do "hands-on" care, such as massage, Reiki, acupressure, etc.?**
  - Some Agencies will offer these extra types of support, while other will not. If any Volunteers provide these kinds of care,

they must first undergo specialized training and pass certification to be able to do so.

- **During a regular "Respite" visit into a Private Residence, how should I respond if the Patient asks me to do something that was not discussed with the Coordinator or with any Family Members; e.g. fetching some food from the refrigerator?**
  - Every situation is unique, but in general during your brief time there You should not do anything that was not anticipated and approved beforehand. The Patient could be diabetic, be on a restricted diet, have problems with swallowing, etc.
- **When going into a facility to visit the Patient one-on-one, what should I do if I find the Patient asleep?**
  - As always, after knocking gently on the door and announcing Yourself, You should approach the Patient quietly. Try to not scare or startle the Individual. Quietly call out the Patient's name several times to see if You get any response. If You do not, and You can confirm the Patient is breathing regularly, You might consider leaving and trying to come back at a different day or time. Sleep or rest can be very important to People struggling with a life-shortening illness.
- **What should I do if the Patient shows no interest in engaging in any planned "Activities" during my visit?**
  - You should always be flexible during each visitation and let the Patient guide the course of any meeting. You ought to have several informal forms of "Activities" You can easily switch to if necessary. So, e.g. if the Patient seems tired and resists doing some arts and crafts project, You may change to simple conversation.
- **Is just watching TV with a Patient sometimes acceptable during visits?**
  - Yes, it is perfectly reasonable if the Patient seems to enjoy the process and Family Members agree. You might watch an old movie that the Family confirms has been a favorite of the

Patient's over the years. Comedy, musicals, preferred series, etc. are all possibilities.

- ***During a regular visit, what should I do if the Patient complains about severe physical pain?***
  - If you are visiting in a Private home setting, You should mention the fact to Family Members. If You are visiting in a facility of some sort, You should relay the information to a staff member. If the pain is severe and unusual, in addition to telling People on site, You should also call your Agency and talk to the on-call Nurse. Visiting Nurses and Home Health Aides may be aware of the changing situation and already be addressing it.

- ***During a regular visit, what should I do if the Patient has declined significantly in either a physical or cognitive way from my last visit?***
  - Personal decline is an inevitable part of the dying process. As You visit the Patient over time, You will be witness to this reality. During your visit, if the Patient appears calm and comfortable, You should simply note the changes in your regular Activity Log. Keep in mind that, in the course of a week, both Nurses and Home Health Aides interact with and assess the Patient's changing conditions.

- ***During a regular visit, what should I do if the Patient appears unusually depressed, anxious or confused?***
  - Again, this may be a normal part of the overall debility of the Patient. You might talk to Family Members or staff members. If the current behaviors and symptoms seem severe or dangerous, You might call the on-call Nurse to discuss the situation. The visiting Nurses and Aides are probably already aware of the circumstances.

- ***What should I do if the Patient dies while I am present?***
  - The practical circumstances are that You will usually never encounter such a situation, except on Vigil Assignments. If this

rare event does occur while You are there, immediately call the Agency.

- ***Can I or should I maintain an on-going friendly relationship with surviving Family Members after the Patient dies?***
  - In general, Hospice Agencies will not encourage or allow such relationships after the final death of the Patient. The Agency will be offering up to 13 months of formal and informal Grief and Bereavement support as required by Medicare Regulations. Volunteers that worked with Patients and Families while the Patient survived are generally discouraged from carrying on any Hospice organizational connection with Survivors. As always, check with your Agency Coordinator concerning these issues.

Virtually all of the above topics will gradually become second nature to You in your work. The more Assignments You take, the more Patients and Family Members You spend time with, the more You study and learn about this challenging field, the more confidence and competence You will develop.

CONCLUSION

▲ ▲ ▲

ALBERT CAMUS' IDEALIZED "METAPHYSICAL REBEL" rejects the consequences implied by death. The consequences are that "everything that dies is ultimately deprived of any inherent meaning" and "if nothing lasts or persists over time, then nothing can possibly be justified". In Hospice Care we side with Camus' Rebel and do everything in our power to insure that these two terrible assertions are wrong.

▲ ▲ ▲

As mentioned before, I have worked as a Hospice Volunteer for over seven years with five separate Agencies and five separate companies in northern California. I have been given the exquisite privilege of sharing the tumultuous journey at life's end with over 200 dying Patients and their Loved Ones. I have worked as a Volunteer in a wide variety of settings, including Private Homes, Assisted Living Facilities, Skilled Nursing Facilities, Dementia Care Wards, Board and Care Units and even Acute-Care Hospitals. I earned a Master's Degree from San Francisco State in 2012 in The Social Work specialty of Gerontology. My specific tract was Quality-of-Life Assessment in End-of-Life Care. I also worked for three years in the Social Services Department in two Skilled Nursing Facilities.

As a Hospice Volunteer, I wrote this Handbook specifically for other Hospice Volunteers. My focus in this first Volume is centered around the Hospice "Friendly Visitor" role and responsibilities. I originally set out to develop a practical guide covering the themes and information I would like to have known when I first started in this complex field. Of course, Agencies strive very hard to prepare and educate their new aspiring Volunteers to be effective in this work. Basic Training parameters are specified by Medicare (and Medicaid). There is also a range of Training Programs available to Agencies to adopt in developing their Volunteers. Beyond these resources, individual Agencies typically develop many of their own Training courses, projects and activities. A natural consequence to this open-ended situation is that Training preparation can vary widely among different Agencies and still comply fully with Federal Regulations. However, each Agency carries a tremendous commitment to Volunteer Training and development. As a new Volunteer, You will naturally benefit tremendously from your own Agency's initial and on-going support. You will likewise find that the various Members of the Hospice Team will be extraordinarily helpful with any questions or issues You might have.

However, the reality is, that there are only so many topics and instructions that can be included within the limited time-frame of any standard Training offered to new Volunteers. This Handbook deals with many practical subjects the Hospice Volunteer will encounter when beginning work with Patients and Family Members. It purposefully goes into great detail about many of these issues.

Each of the six Sections and nineteen Chapters can be separated out and focused on separately. You do not need to go through the book in order nor in any particular sequence. So, if you decide you need to study or go back to review any specific subject matter, You should be able to choose that topic for individual attention.

As a Hospice Volunteer, You will probably start into this challenging field knowing and understanding little about the many ways that Human Beings slip into debility and eventual death. However, with each new Assignment and each next visit, your experience and knowledge will expand. Your capacity for empathy and compassion will grow. If You are willing to be patient with Yourself and persevere, You will gradually become more confident and competent at helping People struggling with the greatest challenge they will ever face. As you continue to endeavor in this terrible and profound experience, one thing will become abundantly clear to You. You will be evolving into the very best version of You.

SUGGESTED READINGS

▲ ▲ ▲

THERE ARE LITERALLY HUNDREDS OF domestic and international books published on the subjects of Hospice and Palliative Care, as well as death and dying in modern society. The following is a concise list of landmark books about these complex subjects. They are listed in no particular order. Hospice Volunteers can and should continue to learn and expand their knowledge even as they grow with each new Assignment and visitation. These important writings should prove vital to the Volunteer's evolution in Human compassion.

- *Handbook for Mortals: Guidance for People Facing Serious Illness*
  (Joanne Lynn – 2011)
- *Changing the Way We Die: Compassionate End of Life Care and the Hospice Movement*
  (Fran Smith – 2013)
- *Modern Death: How Medicine Changed the End of Life*
  (Haider Warraich – 2017)
- *Being Mortal: Medicine and What Matters in the End*
  (Atul Gawande – 2014)
- *The Hospice Choice: In Pursuit of a Peaceful Death*
  (NHPCO – Marcia Lattanzi-Licht – 1998)
- *The Good Death: An Exploration of Dying in America*
  (Ann Neumann – 2017)

- *Living at the End of Life: A Hospice Nurse Addresses the Most Common Questions*
    (Karen Bell – 2011)
- *Sign Posts of Dying: What You Need to Know*
    (Martha Jo Atkins – 2016)
- *A Hospice Guide Book: A Wise Choice Providing Quality Comfort Care Through the EOL...*
    (Curtis Smith – 2012)
- *End-of-Line Care: 20 Common Problems (VITAS)*
    (Barry Weiss et als – 2002)
- *How We Die: Reflections on Life's Final Chapter*
    (Sherwin Nuland – 1993)
- *Final Journeys: A Practical Guide for Bringing Care and Comfort at the End of Life*
- *Final Gifts: Understanding the Special Awareness, Needs and Communications of the Dying*
    (Maggie Callanan – 2009, 2012)
- *Transitions in Dying and Bereavement: A Psychosocial Guide for Hospice and Palliative Care*
    (Victoria House – 2016)
- *Peaceful Passages: A Hospice Nurse's Stories of Dying Well*
    (Janet Wehr – 2015)
- *Dying Well: Peace and Possibilities at the End of Life*
- *The Best Care Possible: A Physician's Quest to Transform Care Through the End of Life*
- *The Four Things that Matter Most: A Book About Living*
    (Ira Byock – 1998, 2013, 2014)
- *From Sun to Sun: A Hospice Nurse Reflects on the Art of Dying*
    (Nina McKissock – 2015)
- *The Needs of the Dying: A Guide for Bringing Hope, Comfort and Love to Life's Final Chapter*
    (David Kessler – 2007)

- *Hospice Whispers: Stories of Life*
        (Carla Cheatham – 2015)
- *Becoming Dead Right: A Hospice Volunteer in Urban Nursing Homes*
        (Frances Parker – 2007)
- *A Few Months to Live: Different Paths to Life's End*
        (Jana Staton – 2001)
- *When Breath Becomes Air*
        (Paul Kalanithi – 2016)
- *On Death and Dying: What the Dying Have to Teach Doctors, Nurses, Clergy and Families*
        (Elizabeth Kubler-Ross – Rev. 2014)
- *Into the Light: Stories About Angelic Visits, Visions of the Afterlife and Pre=Death Experiences*
        (John Lema – 2007)
- *Religious Understandings of a Good Death in Hospice Palliative Care*
        (Harold Coward – 2012)

SUGGESTED RESOURCES

▲ ▲ ▲

THERE ARE MANY FINE NATIONAL and international organizations committed to the advancement of Hospice and Palliative Care ideals. The following is a carefully selected list of specific resources Hospice Volunteers will find enormously helpful in their personal learning and work and growth. These organizations offer training, continuing education, news on current events, legislative agendas, seminars, webinars and guidelines on local and national advocacy issues.

The National Hospice and Palliative Care Organization (nhpco.org)
The Hospice Volunteer Association (hospicevolunteerassociation.org)
Hospice Foundation of America (hospicefoundation.org)
GrowthHouse (growthhouse.org)
American Academy of Hospice and Palliative Medicine (aahpm.org)
International Association for Hospice and Palliative Care (hospicecare.com)
Center to Advance Palliative Care (capc.org)
National Palliative Care Research Center (npcrc.org)

Made in the USA
Las Vegas, NV
12 November 2024

11647648R00103